HEALTHIER LIVES, DIGITALLY ENABLED

Studies in Health Technology and Informatics

International health informatics is driven by developments in biomedical technologies and medical informatics research that are advancing in parallel and form one integrated world of information and communication media and result in massive amounts of health data. These components include genomics and precision medicine, machine learning, translational informatics, intelligent systems for clinicians and patients, mobile health applications, data-driven telecommunication and rehabilitative technology, sensors, intelligent home technology, EHR and patient-controlled data, and Internet of Things.

Studies in Health Technology and Informatics (HTI) series was started in 1990 in collaboration with EU programmes that preceded the Horizon 2020 to promote biomedical and health informatics research. It has developed into a highly visible global platform for the dissemination of original research in this field, containing more than 250 volumes of high-quality works from all over the world.

The international Editorial Board selects publications with relevance and quality for the field. All contributions to the volumes in the series are peer reviewed.

Volumes in the HTI series are submitted for indexing by MEDLINE/PubMed; Web of Science: Conference Proceedings Citation Index – Science (CPCI-S) and Book Citation Index – Science (BKCI-S); Google Scholar; Scopus; EMCare.

Volume 276

Recently published in this series

ISSN 0926-9630 (print)
ISSN 1879-8365 (online)

Healthier Lives, Digitally Enabled

Selected Papers from the Digital Health Institute Summit 2020

Edited by

Mark Merolli

University of Melbourne, Melbourne, Australia

Chris Bain

Monash University, Melbourne, Australia

and

Louise K. Schaper

Australasian Institute of Digital Health, Melbourne, Australia

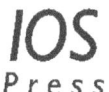

IOS
Press

Amsterdam • Berlin • Washington, DC

ISBN 978-1-64368-168-9 (print)
ISBN 978-1-64368-169-6 (online)
Library of Congress Control Number: 2021935790
doi: 10.3233/SHTI276

Publisher
IOS Press BV
Nieuwe Hemweg 6B
1013 BG Amsterdam
Netherlands
fax: +31 20 687 0019
e-mail: order@iospress.nl

For book sales in the USA and Canada:
IOS Press, Inc.
6751 Tepper Drive
Clifton, VA 20124
USA
Tel.: +1 703 830 6300
Fax: +1 703 830 2300
sales@iospress.com

LEGAL NOTICE

The publisher is not responsible for the use which might be made of the following information.

Preface

2020 has been an unprecedented year in many ways. On top of an already evolving healthcare landscape, nationally and internationally, we have been met with the public and societal health challenge of the COVID-19 pandemic. Not only has this stressed individuals and healthcare systems to their limits but it has also driven an urgent and rapid need to mobilise digital health technology, as well as pressure test digital health in ways and under timeframes not previously imagined. This has its obvious challenges, but it has also created the opportunity for the digital health and informatics community to stand-up and lead. For many, this has meant dealing with digital health projects, such as major electronic medical record (EMR) system implementations at the same time as managing human health. All under very challenging circumstances, while continuing to ensure the safe, effective, and efficient delivery of care in a patient-centred manner. For some others, we have also seen the rapid deployment and uptake of telehealth services, both out of necessity to maintain continuity of care but also to ensure those who need healthcare are still able to access it no matter what the situation or where they are located. Again, it is here that the clinical informatics community has led.

Nationally, the Australasian Institute of Digital Health (AIDH) was launched this year, while all these massive shifts have been occurring all around it. We have continued to be guided under the directives of Australia's National Digital Health Strategy, and recently observed the release of the Australian Digital Health Agency's (ADHA) Workforce and Education Roadmap. This signposts the need to support and deliver on upskilling our health workforce in digital health and informatics. Three key 'horizons' underpin the roadmap, which describes: the use of health record and consumer data, new ways of working with technology, and transformation. There has perhaps been no better time to advocate for our workforce in digital health.

With the workforce in mind, the annual Australian Health Informatics Conference (HIC) represents the coming together of the nation's digital health community to shape the agenda, network, learn, share, and showcase current and future initiatives that support the progression of digital health. Under normal circumstances, HIC provides the place to discuss innovation, digital models of care, data driven decision making, and more. However, and perhaps poetically, this will not look the same in 2020. Considering the COVID-19 pandemic, we will see the emergence of State-led satellite events, coming together with an online feature showcase under the umbrella of the 'Digital Health Institute Summit'. Disruption often drives innovation and having seen the way that the AIDH and the informatics community have embraced digital remote meetings, learning, and social gatherings this year, we have no doubt that the Digital Health Institute Summit will still bring the usual (if not more) vigour, liveliness, and passion for change amongst attendees.

The number of submissions and expressions of interest to present at this year's Summit has been reflective of the passion to continue to drive the digital agenda. We saw overwhelming interest in the form of academic and scientific paper publications. This is reflected in the calibre and breadth that this year's publications demonstrate. This volume of papers reflect highly topical themes across various areas and disciplines. Examples include (but are not limited to): digital health in aged care, mental health,

COVID-19, public health, and workforce. From the digital perspective, we note familiar topics, such as: wearables, mobile health and remote monitoring, interoperability, and data privacy. As well as an increasing appetite for telehealth, automation, bots, and other applications of artificial intelligence.

Like previous years, this year's academic program maintains the same high standard of papers that we know and expect from this conference. All submissions were double blind-peer reviewed by three health informatics experts. We continue to acknowledge the tireless efforts of our volunteer reviewers, without whom, this would not be possible. This thanks extends to the spectacular team at the AIDH, who have been instrumental in supporting this process. 37 papers underwent the initial review. Authors then addressed reviewer feedback and were confirmed by the Scientific Program Committee. What you have here is the culmination of 17 included in this volume. Our sincere congratulations and commendations to the authors of these papers for their contributions to digital health.

Mark Merolli
Chris Bain
Louise K. Schaper

Acknowledgements

The Editors wish to thank the following people for their efforts in reviewing the papers submitted for the Digital Health Institute Summit 2020.

Prof Chris Bain, Monash University
Dr Jen Bichel-Findlay, University of Technology Sydney
A/Prof Ann Borda, University of Melbourne
Ian Bull, Act Health
Dr Kerryn Butler-Henderson FAIDH, University of Tasmania
Dr Elizabeth Cummings FAIDH, University of Tasmania
Khye Davey, East Metropolitan Health Service
Gerardo Luis Dimaguila, Centre for Digital Transformation of Health & School of Computing and Info Systems, The University of Melbourne
Leigh Donoghue, Accenture
Dr Timothy Fazio FAIDH CHIA, The Royal Melbourne Hospital
Andrew Fodor AFAIDH, Epworth Healthcare
Cecily Gilbert, Centre for Digital Transformation of Health
Alan Hamdan, WSLHD
Lis Herbert, Elsevier
A/Prof Inga Hunter FAIDH, Massey University
Chris Mac Manus, Helix, Monash University
Prof Anthony Maeder FAIDH CHIA, Flinders University
Greg Moran CHIA, Australasian Institute of Digital Health
Dr Abraham Oshni Alvandi, Monash
Matthew Painter, North Metropolitan Health Service
Jeremy Roach FAIDH, Jeremy Roach Pty Ltd
Philip Robinson FAIDH, Acrobatic Consulting Services
Angela Ryan FAIDH, Australian Digital Health Agency
Beth Sperring, Royal Perth Hospital
Susan Stemp, Cairns and Hinterland Hospital and Health Service
Richard Taggart FAIDH CHIA, Sydney Local Health District
Louise Van Der Kraan, DXC Technology
Peter Williams FAIDH CHIA, Oracle
Yvonne Zardins, Telstra Health

Contents

Healthier Lives, Digitally Enabled
M. Merolli et al. (Eds.)
doi:10.3233/SHTI210002

Bring-Your-Own-Device Usage Trends in Australian Hospitals – A National Survey

Tafheem Ahmad WANI [a,1], Antonette MENDOZA [a] and Kathleen GRAY [b]

[a] *School of Computing and Information Systems, The University of Melbourne*
[b] *Centre for Digital Transformation of Health, The University of Melbourne*

Abstract. Background: Healthcare is among the leading industries which drives the use of personal devices for work purposes (BYOD). However, allowing BYOD for healthcare workers comes at a cost, as it puts sensitive information assets such as patient data residing on personal devices at risk of potential data breaches. Objective: Previous review of the literature has highlighted the dearth of empirical studies in hospital settings regarding BYOD usage. As such, this paper aims to report BYOD usage trends in Australian hospitals through a national survey, first of its kind in Australia. Methods: An anonymous survey was conducted online among health IT personnel, asking them about their experiences about BYOD usage in their hospitals. 28 responses were collected based on public Australian hospitals, which included 21 hospital groups and 7 standalone hospitals, likely to represent more than 100 hospitals in total. Survey responses were quantitatively analysed through descriptive statistical analysis and cross tabulation. Results: BYOD is allowed in majority of the hospitals, and among all major staff groups, with doctors being the leading group. Participants ranked reasons for allowing BYOD, and most of them were related to improvement in clinical productivity, efficiency and mobility for clinical staff. Challenges were generally related to data security such as patient data breaches and compliance with data security laws, according to them. More than two thirds of hospitals had a cybersecurity officer employed, and CIOs were the most dominant group who held responsibility for managing BYOD within the hospital. Conclusion: This paper provides a starting point for better understanding of BYOD usage in a complex healthcare environment based on empirical evidence, one which highlights the security-usability conundrum, confirming previous literature themes.

Keywords. BYOD, bring-your-own-device, cybersecurity, health, hospital, privacy

1. Introduction

'Bring-your-own-device' or BYOD is a common practice in workplaces, where employees use their personal mobile devices such as smartphones, tablets, laptops for carrying out professional or work-related tasks [1]. Healthcare is one of the leading industries driving BYOD usage [2]. Healthcare professionals typically perform a range of work-related tasks using their personal devices: accessing electronic medical records, clinical documentation, photography, diagnostic or drug information results, and for communication or collaboration with fellow staff or patients [3, 4] . Not only does BYOD improve the productivity and efficiency of clinicians, it also enhances their mobility and allows them to provide patient care within and outside hospital or clinic workplaces [5]. For example, the COVID-19 pandemic has created an upsurge in use of BYOD by hospital staff for purposes such as telehealth consultations and remote work [6, 7].

---

[1] Corresponding Author, Tafheem Ahmad Wani, School of Computing and Information Systems, The University of Melbourne, Parkville, Victoria, Australia 3010, E-mail: twani@student.unimelb.edu.au.

However, BYOD is a major challenge for hospitals due to data security concerns and is seen as one of the biggest healthcare IT challenges [8]. Healthcare sees the greatest number of data breaches of all industries, not only in Australia but world-wide, with BYOD being a major reason [9, 10, 11]. Hospitals typically don't have any control on the number and type of devices their employees use, nor their device usage behaviour, which increases the risk of data breaches, including patient data. Each device added to the hospital network is a potential cybersecurity threat [12]. Also, hospital compliance with patient data privacy laws is difficult in a BYOD environment [9, 13]. Continuing the COVID-19 example, the increase in remote work among healthcare workers during the pandemic has led to several data breaches where BYOD was a major cause [6, 7, 14].

Previous reviews of both academic and grey literature identified social, technical and managerial issues associated with BYOD usage [12, 15]. However, they showed that there is a dearth of empirical studies of BYOD usage in healthcare settings, especially in Australia, given its unique health IT context as well as a different set of laws concerning healthcare data breaches [12, 16, 17]. Hence, this paper reports on actual BYOD usage trends in Australian hospitals. Information about access obtained via BYOD, socio-technical security measures, benefits and further analysis was also asked as part of this survey, but this would be covered in a future publication due to this paper's size limits.

2. Methodology

A national Australian survey recruited volunteers among health IT personnel with an overview knowledge of BYOD usage within their respective hospitals. The survey asked questions about participants' experiences with BYOD practices in mid-to large size hospitals, with human research ethics approval (Ethics ID: 1955486.1) obtained from the University of Melbourne. Preliminary research based on literature review and a conceptual framework developed by the authors was used to frame survey questions [12, 15, 18]. The survey was setup online using the Qualtrics survey platform. Only anonymous data was collected, with no information requested which could individually identify a participant or a hospital. This was done to make sure that sensitivities about potentially pinpointing a specific organisation's practices or gaps are carefully recognised. The survey used Qualtrics IP filtering to avoid duplication of responses.

The survey was promoted through webinars and social media groups (particularly associated with cyber security) of professional organisations such as Australian Institute of Digital Health (AIDH), Health Information and Management Systems Society (HIMSS) and platforms such as LinkedIn. It was also sent to all state government health CIOs or people in similar positions for information and circulation. Responses were collected during a four-month period from March to June 2020. An anonymous link was used for distribution, which was carefully circulated to avoid duplication.

28 responses were collected from participants based in public hospitals from four Australian states. 21 survey responses were based on BYOD practices in hospital groups, while 7 concerned standalone hospitals. Given that each hospital group comprises an average of 3-7 hospitals in Australia, the number of hospitals reflected in the survey is likely more than 100 – compared to a total of 693 public hospitals in Australia [19]. Survey questions were analysed quantitatively through descriptive statistical analysis and cross tabulation, using Qualtrics analysis platform, as well as Excel. The results presented here provide an initial picture of BYOD usage in Australian hospitals.

3. Results

3.1. Individual and Hospital Characteristics

The survey was completed by IT personnel with different designations including Chief Information Officer (CIO), Chief Information Security Officer (CISO), IT Director, IT Manager, IT Infrastructure Manager, and Information Security Manager. 11 participants (39.29%) had worked in the hospital or hospital group about which they supplied information for up to 5 years, 9 participants (32.14%) for 6-10 years, and 8 participants (28.57%) for more than 10 years.

The hospitals about which information was supplied, were diverse. With respect to their principal location which participants described, 8 responses (28.57%) were based on hospitals or hospital groups in inner city locations, 8 responses (28.57%) were suburban hospital or hospital group based, 8 responses (28.57%) based on regional centre hospitals or hospital groups and 4 responses (14.29%) based on hospital groups having both a metropolitan and regional presence. With respect to staff size, most surveys reflected large hospital settings. 24 responses (85.71%) were based on hospitals or hospital groups with staff over 1000, 3 responses (10.71%) with 500-1000 staff size and 1 response (3.57%) based on a hospital organisation with staff size less than 500.

3.2. BYOD Usage Trends

3.2.1. BYOD Usage Permission

22 participants (78.57%) said that BYOD was allowed in their hospital/hospital group. Only 5 participants (17.86%) said that BYOD wasn't allowed. One participant (3.57%) said that the policy regarding allowing use of BYOD was not clearly specified to the staff. Out of the 5 participants who said BYOD wasn't allowed in their hospital/hospital group, 4 participants (80%) were unsure if it will be allowed in the next 2 years, whereas 1 participant (20%) said that it won't be allowed even after that. No-one was certain that BYOD would be allowed in the next 2 years. Cross tabulation analysis further reveals that BYOD is allowed in majority of metropolitan hospitals and in hospitals with a large staff size, as opposed to regional hospitals. Specific details on exact distribution across different types of hospitals can be found in Table 1.

Table 1. Cross tabulation analysis on BYOD usage permission based on location and staff size

Hospital Type	Total Count	Whether BYOD Allowed or Not		
Principal Location		Yes	No	Not Sure
Inner City	8	8 (100%)	0 (0%)	0 (0%)
Suburban	8	8 (100%)	0 (0%)	0 (0%)
Regional Centre	8	3 (37.5%)	4 (50%)	1 (12.5%)
Other	4	3 (75%)	1 (25%)	0 (0%)
Staff Size				
Less than 500	1	1 (100%)	0 (0%)	0 (0%)
Between 500 - 1000	3	2 (66.67%)	1 (33.33%)	0 (0%)
More than 1000	24	19 (79.17%)	4 (16.67%)	1 (4.16%)
GRAND TOTAL	**28**	**22 (78.57%)**	**5 (17.86%)**	**1 (3.57%)**

3.2.2. BYOD Usage by Staff

Clinical, IT and administrative staff were allowed to use BYOD among the hospital/hospital groups which allowed it. Out of 23 hospitals / groups which allowed BYOD, 21 (91.30%) allowed BYOD for doctors and 20 (86.96%) allowed it for IT staff. This was followed by administrative and clerical staff - 17 (73.91%), nurses - 16 (69.57%), diagnostic and allied health professionals - 16 (69.57%) and domestic and other personal care staff - 11 (47.83%).

3.2.3. Reasons for Allowing and Disallowing BYOD

Participants were asked to rank reasons for allowing BYOD in hospitals/hospital groups, based on a number of options given in the survey. According to majority of the participants, improvement in clinical productivity or efficiency among staff was the topmost reason for allowing BYOD in their hospital, with 14 participants (60.87%) out of 23 ranking it number 1. Based on average ranking score, this was followed by: improvement in employee satisfaction (ranked 2), making teleworking easier (ranked 3), saving money (ranked 4), difficulty in enforcing bans on BYOD use (ranked 5) and reducing device procurement workload on IT (ranked 6).

Among hospitals/hospital groups not allowing BYOD, 3 participants (60%) out of 5 selected patient data breaches as the topmost reason for not allowing BYOD. Lesser reasons included IT management/administration overhead (ranked 2), compliance with healthcare data privacy laws (ranked 3), security management costs (ranked 4), reimbursement for staff (ranked 5), inadvertent mixing of private and professional data (ranked 6) and regulating user behaviour (ranked 7).

3.2.4. Major Challenges Related to BYOD

For hospitals or hospital groups allowing BYOD, participants were asked to rank challenges related to BYOD, based on a number of options given in the survey. The top ranked challenge was compliance with healthcare data privacy laws, with 10 participants (43.48%) out of 23 ranking this as number 1. This was followed by patient data breaches (ranked 2), regulating user behaviour (ranked 3), security management costs (ranked 4), IT management/administration overhead (ranked 5), reimbursement for staff (ranked 6) and inadvertent mixing of private and professional data (ranked 7).

3.2.5. BYOD Program Ownership

Program ownership refers to allocating the overall responsibility of a particular program to a unit or person for better accountability. 21 participants (95.45%) out of 22 whose organisations allowed BYOD said that their hospitals had allocated the overall responsibility for the program to a staff role. 19 participants (90.47%) said that the CIO held ownership of the BYOD program, 1 participant (4.76%) said that the CTO was the owner and 1 participant (4.76%) said that the CEO was responsible for the program.

3.2.6. Cybersecurity Personnel Employed in the Hospital/Hospital Group

19 participants (67.86%) said that their hospital/hospital group had a dedicated cybersecurity officer for managing information security affairs. Further distribution is provided in Table 2 using cross-tabulation analysis.

Table 2. Cross tabulation analysis of whether cybersecurity personnel employed or not.

Hospital Characteristic	Total Count	Whether Cybersecurity Personnel Employed	
		Yes	No
Principal Location			
Inner City	8	6 (75%)	2 (25%)
Suburban	8	6 (75%)	2 (25%)
Regional Centre	8	5 (62.5%)	3 (37.5%)
Other	4	2 (50%)	2 (50%)
Staff Size			
Less than 500	1	1 (100%)	0 (0%)
Between 500 - 1000	3	1 (33.33%)	2 (66.67%)
More than 1000	24	17 (70.83%)	7 (29.17%)
GRAND TOTAL	**28**	**19 (67.86%)**	**9 (32.14%)**

4. Discussion

The hospital industry in Australia follows the global trend, as survey responses suggest that BYOD is allowed by majority of the hospitals and across all staff groups. The survey findings also indicate that the familiarity and convenience of using personal devices for work by clinicians is thought to boost their clinical productivity and save their time. Out of the different clinician groups, BYOD usage was reported to be particularly high among doctors; this may be due to the nature of a doctor's work across multiple hospitals and other clinical settings. On the other hand, nurses may be more strongly affiliated with a single hospital, and BYOD usage may be constrained by more interaction with in-hospital record-keeping systems, or greater infection control considerations. Further research is under way involving clinical participants, to shed more light on whether a differential approach may be required for different clinical roles, when choosing whether to allow BYOD and/or what services to allow.

The survey suggests that the topmost issues associated with BYOD use relate to security, which includes patient data breaches and non-compliance with data privacy laws, confirming themes from the literature. The same reason was quoted by participants for not allowing BYOD. The data also implies that regional hospitals may also face the additional challenge of lack of budget to maintain cybersecurity requirements. This is a huge concern for hospitals as BYOD is a major contributor for health data breaches. It is also becoming difficult for hospitals to comply with strict government regulations as highlighted previously. This might be the reason that it was ranked as the number 1 challenge concerning BYOD use.

This indicates the need for security and usability balance, as the authors have highlighted previously [12, 15]. To address this challenge, hospitals not only need to leverage their existing IT security technologies, but also to have BYOD policies and training programs for staff which can provide them guidance for productive, flexible and safe use of BYOD to ensure proper compliance. Hospitals where ownership of BYOD programs is the responsibility of the CIO, or of a dedicated cybersecurity officer, indicate steps in the right direction.

This survey is first of its kind to be reported in Australia. Its major limitation is that there may be a degree of imprecision associated with data collection, as it was very important to elicit anonymous responses from senior hospital insiders, without compromising reputations or further jeopardising privacy of these organisations. Features such as automatic IP filtering and survey protection was used to avoid this. Also, the diversity of the nature of hospital settings represented in this survey also makes it unlikely or minimal. Further, it does not reflect practices in the private hospital sector, or in primary and community healthcare organisations. This paper presents only the first part of a larger study by the authors exploring the people, policy and technology factors in balancing the risks and benefits of BYOD in hospitals. Further research will provide a deeper analysis of the technical, social and managerial aspects of BYOD security.

Overall, this work contributes a new understanding of BYOD in Australian hospitals. It raises the profile of this ubiquitous and pragmatic aspect of health information technology, and therefore provides the start of a roadmap for improving careful and responsible BYOD use.

References

[1]   D. Arregui, S. Maynard, and A. Ahmad, "Mitigating BYOD information security risks," 2015. Available: http://minerva-access.unimelb.edu.au/handle/11343/56627.
[2]   "BYOD (Bring Your Own Device) Market Analysis, Market Size, Application Analysis, Regional Outlook, Competitive Strategies and Forecasts, 2016 To 2024," Hexa Research, Dec. 2016.
[3]   A. Nerminathan, A. Harrison, M. Phelps, S. Alexander, and K. M. Scott, "Doctors' use of mobile devices in the clinical setting: a mixed methods study," *Intern. Med. J.*, vol. 47, no. 3, pp. 291–298, 2017, doi: 10.1111/imj.13349.
[4]   M. Moreau and G. Paré, "Early clinical management of severe burn patients using telemedicine: a pilot study protocol," *Pilot Feasibility Stud.*, vol. 6, no. 1, p. 93, Jul. 2020, doi: 10.1186/s40814-020-00637-7.
[5]   J. Williams, "Left to Their Own Devices How Healthcare Organizations Are Tackling the BYOD Trend,"
[6]   *Biomed. Instrum. Technol.*, vol. 48, no. 5, p. 327, Sep. 2014.
[7]   Bitglass, "Bitglass 2020 BYOD Report: Remote Work Drives BYOD, but Security Not Keeping Pace," 2020.   https://www.bitglass.com/press-releases/bitglass-2020-byod-report-remote-work-drives-byod-but-security-not-keeping-pace
[8]   J. Davis, "Must-Have Telehealth, Remote Work Privacy and Security for COVID-19," *HealthITSecurity*, Mar. 31, 2020.
[9]   J. L. Schiff, "The 4 biggest healthcare IT headaches," *CIO*, May 23, 2017. https://www.cio.com/article/3197698/healthcare/the-4-biggest-healthcare-it-headaches.html
[10] L. Coventry and D. Branley, "Cybersecurity in healthcare: A narrative review of trends, threats and ways forward," *Maturitas*, vol. 113, pp. 48–52, Jul. 2018, doi: 10.1016/j.maturitas.2018.04.008.
[11] J. Davis, "Health Sector Most Targeted by Hackers, Breach Costs Rise to $17.76B," *HealthITSecurity*, Jun. 09, 2020.
[12] OAIC, "Notifiable Data Breaches scheme 12-month insights report," 2019. [Online]. Available: https://www.oaic.gov.au/privacy/notifiable-data-breaches/notifiable-data-breaches-statistics/notifiable-data-breaches-scheme-12month-insights-report/.
[13] T. A. Wani, A. Mendoza, and K. Gray, "Hospital Bring-Your-Own-Device Security Challenges and Solutions: Systematic Review of Gray Literature," *JMIR MHealth UHealth*, vol. 8, no. 6, p. e18175, 2020, doi: 10.2196/18175.
[14] E. Snell, "4 Key Concerns in Healthcare Mobile Security Options," *HealthITSecurity*, Aug. 17, 2017.
[15] J. Davis, "Remote Attacks on Cloud Service Targets Rose 630% Amid COVID-19," HealthITSecurity, Jun. 2020. Available: https://healthitsecurity.com/news/remote-attacks-on-cloud-service-targets-rose-630-amid-covid-19.
[16] T. A. Wani, A. Mendoza, and K. Gray, "BYOD in Hospitals-Security Issues and Mitigation Strategies," in *Proceedings of the Australasian Computer Science Week Multiconference*, New York, NY, USA, 2019, p. 25:1–25:10, doi: 10.1145/3290688.3290729.
[17] J. E. Moyer, "Managing Mobile Devices in Hospitals: A Literature Review of BYOD Policies and Usage."
[18] *J. Hosp. Librariansh.*, vol. 13, no. 3, pp. 197–208, Jul. 2013, doi: 10.1080/15323269.2013.798768.
[19] N. Zahadat, P. Blessner, T. Blackburn, and B. A. Olson, "BYOD security engineering: A framework and its analysis," *Comput. Secur.*, vol. 55, pp. 81–99, Nov. 2015, doi: 10.1016/j.cose.2015.06.011.
[20] S. Schlarman, "The People, Policy, Technology (PPT) Model: Core Elements of the Security Process,"
[21] *Inf. Syst. Secur.*, vol. 10, no. 5, pp. 1–6, 2006, doi: 10.1201/1086/43315.10.5.20011101/31719.6.
[22] AIHW, "Hospital resources 2017–18: Australian hospital statistics, At a glance," AIHW, 2019. [Online]. Available: https://www.aihw.gov.au/reports/hospitals/hospital-resources-2017-18-ahs/contents/at-a-glance.

Healthier Lives, Digitally Enabled
M. Merolli et al. (Eds.)

7

doi:10.3233/SHTI210003

Caregivers' Perspectives on Privacy in Aged Care Monitoring Devices

Sami ALKHATIB [a,b], Jenny WAYCOTT [a], George BUCHANAN [a],
Marthie GROBLER [b] and Shuo WANG [b]

[a] *School of Computing and Information Systems, University of Melbourne, Australia*
[b] *CSIRO's Data61, Melbourne, Australia*

Abstract. As people move into advanced old age, they may experience cognitive impairments and frailty, making it difficult for them to live without support from others. Caregivers might decide to use aged care monitoring devices (ACMDs) to support older adults under their care. However, these devices raise privacy concerns as they collect and share sensitive data from the older adult's private life in order to provide monitoring capabilities. This study involved interviewing formal and informal caregivers who used/may use ACMDs to investigate their views on privacy. The study found that although caregivers consider protecting older adults' privacy important, they may overlook privacy in order to gain benefits from ACMDs. We argue that ACMD developers should simplify privacy terms and conditions so that caregivers can make well-informed decisions when deciding to use the device. They also should consider providing users with flexible privacy settings so that users can decide what data to collect, whom to share it with and when.

Keywords. aged care, caregiving, privacy, monitoring

1. Introduction

As people move into advanced old age, they may experience cognitive impairments and frailty, making it difficult for them to live without receiving support from others. Informal caregivers (e.g. family members) and/or formal caregivers (e.g. paid aged care workers) may be required to check on and assist older adults under their care. This can be challenging and a source of considerable distress for caregivers, in particular when they support older adults who require frequent attention [5].

Aged Care Monitoring Devices (ACMDs) support older adults living alone at home or in residential care facilities. These devices collect older adults' health and wellbeing information and share it with caregivers using the Internet. ACMDs provide caregivers with peace of mind by ensuring they will be informed whenever older adults need help [12]. Despite the expected benefits from using ACMDs, these devices pose privacy challenges as they collect and share older adults' personal details with others [1]. Caregivers using ACMDs may be able to know details from older adults' lives that might be deemed as sensitive. Moreover, ACMD service providers may use the collected data to create behavioural and health records in order to use them for unintended purposes (e.g. marketing and research) without older adults' consent.

Although caregivers might decide to use monitoring devices to help them provide better support to older adults [16], previous studies found that older adults may reject using these devices due to their privacy concerns [2]. However, only a few studies have investigated caregivers' perspectives in the use of ACMDs and whether older adults' privacy is one of their concerns [18]. This paper addresses this gap by exploring caregivers' privacy perception in the use of ACMDs. The findings will inform ACMD developers about caregivers' privacy concerns to help them create monitoring devices that support older adults' and retain their privacy at the same time.

2. Study Aims

The role of the caregivers in deciding to use ACMDs, particularly for older adults experiencing cognitive impairment, is crucial [10], [14]. However, there is limited understanding of how caregivers view of privacy in the use of ACMDs. This study aims to fill this knowledge gap by conducting in-depth interviews with informal and formal caregivers, to gain insights into how caregivers perceive privacy in the use of ACMDs and their privacy concerns that need to be addressed.

3. Method

We conducted an interview study with 12 caregivers (8 informal and 4 formal caregivers) to gain insights into how caregivers perceive privacy in ACMDs. Although 12 is a small sample size, this study aimed to gain in-depth insights rather than broad generalisations. Further, the sample size aligns with other similar studies. For instance, Caine [4] and Marshall et al. [12] found in their review studies that a considerable number of computing science empirical studies rely on around 12 participants to provide findings. To recruit participants, we contacted aged care facilities, home care service providers and ACMD companies to nominate informal/ formal caregivers as potential interviewees. We then contacted the nominated caregivers via email to inform them about the study and schedule an interview if they were interested.

Out of the 12 participants, 3 informal and 4 formal caregivers were using ACMDs, 3 informal caregivers had used ACMDs previously (e.g. GPS trackers and fall detectors). Two informal caregivers never used an ACMD. In this paper, all participants are anonymised and referred to by IP1, 2, 3 etc. for informal caregivers and FP1, 2, 3 etc. for formal caregivers.

Interviews were semi-structured; we used a set of questions as a guide, but sometimes we asked other questions to further explore interesting answers provided by the participants. The questions were open-ended so that participants could provide as much detail as they wanted to. Questions included: "what type of information do you prefer to be collected by using a monitoring device?" and "what do you know about privacy policies associated with these devices?". In addition, we read a scenario [8] based on the "Uninvited Guests" video by Superflux [17], which depicts Thomas, a man in his 70s who received ACMDs from his children to monitor diet, activities and sleep. The scenario was used to provoke discussion about privacy and to better understand what sort of information participants felt comfortable collecting through ACMDs, when and with whom they prefer to share this information.

The interpretive approach was implemented to make sense of the interview transcripts. This involves gaining insights about the phenomenon explored by interpreting the meanings people assign to it [19]. Following an interpretive approach corresponds with the aim of our study of getting a better understanding of caregivers' views on privacy in the use of ACMDs.

4. Findings

In this section, we discuss privacy perceptions and views in the use of ACMDs that caregivers in this study had: 1) benefits versus risks, 2) limited data sharing and 3) using ACMDs, the decision is older adults' too.

4.1. Benefits Versus Risks

Participants indicated that using ACMDs should be well-justified whether they are used to monitor older adults living in their home or in an aged care facility. For instance, IP1 said *"There has to be [for using ACMDs] a very clear justification or a rationale for it"*.

In order to justify using ACMDs, participants emphasised that the benefits of using these devices should outweigh any privacy risks associated with them. However, we noted that different participants had different views on what they perceived as a benefit that outweighs privacy risks. For instance, IP5 suggested that any type of monitoring is accepted as long as it extends the ability of older adults to remain in their home as they age: *"That's a lesser of the evils [losing privacy] of putting mum monitored. It's my job to make sure that we respect it [her privacy] as much as practically possible. So, it's for filling her ambition in staying home and be supported"*. IP7, however, emphasised that although using ACMDs may enable older adults to live independently in their home, uncontrolled monitoring - by knowing personal details about older adults under their care without any restrictions - is unacceptable and likened it to surveillance. For instance, IP7 commented on Thomas's scenario and said: *"I'm extremely uncomfortable with what you've just said. It's George Orwell"*.

Other participants drew links between the expected benefits of using ACMDs and the type of data that these devices will collect and share. They pointed out that ACMDs should only monitor health and wellbeing information required to mitigate negative consequences related to specific concerns. This should be decided based on the current needs of older adults and any known previous health or wellbeing indicators related to previously identified issues. As an example: *"The one device I did use was a tracker, so that I could tell where he was. He did wander a period of time, so I did use that on several occasions"* (IP4). One type of information that most of the participants agreed will be beneficial to monitor was detecting falls. Falls are common among older people and can have severe consequences. FP2 said: *"Smart mat, if they [aged care residents] are at high risk of falls, that will alert us when they're trying to come out of the bed"*.

Similarly, formal caregivers noted that ACMDs can assist them in their work, particularly to monitor older adults who are experiencing cognitive problems. This helps caregivers ensure that older adults get the necessary treatment and remain safe. For instance, FP2 said: *"Well, the wandering alarm, we really needed it because we have residents that are at high risk of absconding. We had already few situations where they actually got away and absconded"*. FP4 provided another example of a potential use to help provide the right treatment and said: *"They've put her [resident] on a Coloxyl [treat constipation] morning and night. She might go to the toilet, but she doesn't remember and tells them that she hasn't been and so then they give her something [Coloxyl]"*.

Participants indicated that they will accept using ACMD if they perceive the benefits to outweigh privacy risks. Describing this relation, IP5 said, *"Quite frankly, it's a risk benefit equation. So, what's the benefit I'm getting from doing this? And what's the risk associated with it? If I'm not going to have any risk, I'm not going to get any benefit".*

4.2. Limited Data Sharing

Participants emphasised that ACMDs should only share information whenever these devices detect concerning indicators that require immediate intervention (e.g. falls). Otherwise, sharing a limited number of wellbeing status reports should be sufficient as long as these reports confirm that older adults are doing fine. For instance, IP5 said: *"Emergencies! You don't want to know day-to-day activities. One message per day is good, it's another way of monitoring how she's [mother living alone] going".*

Although formal caregivers prefer to only receive alarms for emergency situations, they noted that it is their responsibility to check data collected by ACMDs regularly. Formal caregivers indicated that they are guided by their workplace processes. For instance, FP2 noted that she has to regularly check a monitor to see a visual of reports from monitoring devices from residents' rooms: *"Probably ... we do it every two hours".*

Most participants indicated that the collected information should only be shared with certain people. IP1 said: *"It's only to significant people, relevant people and only the relevant information. I would say it's the person who is in charge of care".* Participants were worried about sharing collected information with unintended parties as this may lead to unintended uses such as for marketing campaigns. IP4 said: *"That does worry me that somebody there knows what you're thinking, and tracking what you're looking at, and then applying marketing, and advertising, not appropriately"* IP5 noted that it is unacceptable to share older adults' collected data with any third-parties. IP5 justified this by indicating that users pay money to buy a monitoring device and are not providing data in exchange for a free service, as is the case with Facebook. As a solution, IP5 suggested that companies should consider optional privacy settings; customers need to be able to determine with whom to share their data and for what purposes. For instance, ACMD users might want their data to be used for other purposes in exchange for reduced costs: *"So they say, 'we'll harvest your information and sell it, I will give you a reduction in your price of the unit or here's the price of the unit and it's completely secure and private your choice'.".*

4.3. Using ACMDs, the Decision is Older Adults' Too

Most of the participants emphasised the importance of older adults' consent when using ACMD. They believe that older adults should be aware that they are monitored by these devices and provide well-informed consent before using them. This means not to impose using ACMDs on older adults and to discuss details with them about the purpose of the device before using it. For instance, IP2 commented on Thomas's scenario and said: *"If he is happy to have his daughter know those things [monitoring him], then that's fine. But if she is imposing that on dad without his consent or his agreement maybe not... And it needs to be an open consent, not a grudging one".*

Although formal caregivers indicated that they discuss the purpose of new ACMD with their residents, they pointed out that residents of aged care facilities may not always be able to provide consent. FP2 emphasised that caregivers are obliged to protect their residents by taking any necessary action(s) based on their specific needs: *"They have no* choice sometimes, so they have to accept it. We do explain to them why they are having the mat [to detect if residents get out of bed]. Some residents are a bit resistive to it. They'd be like, it's my right if I want to get up and walk, I can do it".

However, two informal caregivers who have older relatives in residential care noted that these facilities should not take older adults' consent for granted whenever they use ACMDs to monitor them. They indicated that there are residents in aged care facilities who are not capable of making decisions by themselves and may need assistance to decide. IP1 said, *"Because they can't give informed consent, it shouldn't be assumed that it's okay. It's not okay if a person can't give a consent".* IP1 therefore emphasised that proxies - who are responsible for answering questions on older adults' behalf, particularly regarding health and care services [3] - should be consulted before using ACMDs, *"I would object strongly to any device being used without discussions with me and without my approval, because I speak for her [wife in residential care]".* Both participants indicated that privacy decisions should be respectful. Caregivers need to be well-informed about any ACMD to be used and carefully consider what is proper in terms of privacy based on older adults' circumstances. IP6 said: *"I think privacy comes under to me, it would be, how would you wish to be treated if you were receiving care".*

To be well-informed about what happens with the data collected by ACMDs, it is necessary to read privacy policies provided with these devices. Although privacy policies provide users with details on how service providers will handle, protect and use users' data [6], we found that only two participants consider(ed) reading privacy policies and terms and conditions before using these devices. IP8 said: *"I'm the sort of person who reads all 69 pages of a document that might handle something because I want to know whether it was relevant".* Other participants indicated that they simply choose to accept terms and conditions without reading them. IP5 said, *"You know what!? You just flagged something that I completely ignored. We would tick the box where you just agree to terms and conditions that we haven't even read".*

Participants reported two main reasons for not reading ACMD privacy policies: 1) privacy policies are too long and use technical jargon that is difficult to understand 2) some caregivers may need to use a monitoring device regardless of its privacy risks. IP8 said: *"I think it's related to 2 things; the privacy policies are too long and too complicated, and the thing is that we just want to get this working down as you know".*

5. Discussion and Conclusion

We found that all participants in this study were aware that older adults' privacy will be affected by using ACMDs. Participants noted that decisions about using ACMDs should balance between benefits provided and privacy risks. This is in line with findings from previous studies such as Robinson et al. [15] and Landau et al. [10]. Participants therefore emphasised that any ACMD should strictly limit any collection and sharing of older adults' data. For instance, fall detectors were considered beneficial by all participants as falls are common between elderly people and may cause serious injuries [9]. However, only caregivers who are directly responsible for older adults' wellbeing should receive alerts about falls so they can act to avoid negative consequences.

Furthermore, most of the participants refused to impose using ACMDs on older adults. They emphasised that details on the purpose of the device should be discussed with older adults so they can provide a well-informed consent before using the device. Participants were mostly concerned about privacy as non-invasiveness, nonintrusiveness and non-obtrusiveness over information privacy in the use of ACMDs [7]. Only few participants and due to the complexity of privacy policies, were interested in knowing about information privacy including privacy protection measurements (i.e. protections against technical issues such as hacking) applied by service providers. Interestingly, this includes knowing whether the collected data will be shared with third parties and the purposes that the data will be used for before they start using ACMDs.

Caregivers play an important role in influencing older adults' decisions on using monitoring devices [14]. We noticed that caregivers might overlook privacy out of necessity, in particular for those who want to avoid a previous bad experience (e.g. fall or wandering) from happening again in the future. We therefore argue that ACMD developers should consider various older adults' and caregivers' perspectives in relation to privacy such as what data to collect, whom to share it with and when. This requires simplifying privacy notices in terms and conditions by making them short and simple to avoid overwhelming caregivers with unnecessary details. Moreover, developers should consider offering ACMD users different privacy settings so that users are able to tailor their own preferences based on their needs [11].

References

[1]   Alkhatib, S., Waycott, J., & Buchanan, G. (2019, August). Privacy in Aged Care Monitoring Devices (ACMD): The Developers' Perspective. In Digital Health: Changing the Way Healthcare is Conceptualised and Delivered: Selected Papers from the 27th Australian National Health Informatics Conference (HIC 2019) (Vol. 266, p. 7). IOS Press.
[2]   Astell, A. J., McGrath, C., & Dove, E. (2019). 'That's for old so and so's!': does identity influence older adults' technology adoption decisions?. Ageing & Society, 1-27.
[3]   Caiels, J., Rand, S., Crowther, T., Collins, G., & Forder, J. (2019). Exploring the views of being a proxy from the perspective of unpaid carers and paid carers: developing a proxy version of the Adult Social Care Outcomes Toolkit (ASCOT). BMC health services research, 19(1), 201.
[4]   Caine, K. (2016, May). Local standards for sample size at CHI. In Proceedings of the 2016 CHI conference on human factors in computing systems (pp. 981-992).
[5]   Grossi, E., Lucchi, E., Gentile, S., Trabucchi, M., Bellelli, G., & Morandi, A. (2019). Preliminary investigation of predictors of distress in informal caregivers of patients with delirium superimposed on dementia. Aging clinical and experimental research, 1-6.
[6]   Henze, M., Hummen, R., & Wehrle, K. (2013, May). The cloud needs cross-layer data handling annotations. In 2013 IEEE Security and Privacy Workshops (pp. 18-22). IEEE.
[7]   Ienca, M., Wangmo, T., Jotterand, F., Kressig, R. W., & Elger, B. (2018). Ethical design of intelligent assistive technologies for dementia: a descriptive review. Science and engineering ethics, 24(4), 1035-1055.
[8]   Krupp, M. M., Rueben, M., Grimm, C. M., & Smart, W. D. (2017, August). A focus group study of privacy concerns about telepresence robots. In 2017 26th IEEE International Symposium on Robot and Human Interactive Communication (RO-MAN) (pp. 1451-1458). IEEE.
[9]   Larizza, M. F., Zukerman, I., Bohnert, F., Busija, L., Bentley, S. A., Russell, R. A., & Rees, G. (2014). In-home monitoring of older adults with vision impairment: exploring patients', caregivers' and professionals' views. Journal of the American Medical Informatics Association, 21(1), 56-63.
[10] Landau, R., Auslander, G. K., Werner, S., Shoval, N., & Heinik, J. (2010). Families' and professional caregivers' views of using advanced technology to track people with dementia. Qualitative health research, 20(3), 409-419.
[11] Mahoney, D. F. (2011). An evidence-based adoption of technology model for remote monitoring of elders' daily activities. Ageing international, 36(1), 66-81.
[12] Marshall, B., Cardon, P., Poddar, A., & Fontenot, R. (2013). Does sample size matter in qualitative research? A review of qualitative interviews in IS research. Journal of Computer Information Systems, 54(1), 11-22.
[13] McCabe, L., & Innes, A. (2013). Supporting safe walking for people with dementia: User participation in the development of new technology. Gerontechnology, 12(1), 4-15.

[14] Peek, S. T., Luijkx, K. G., Rijnaard, M. D., Nieboer, M. E., van der Voort, C. S., ... & Wouters, E. J. (2016). Older adults' reasons for using technology while aging in place. Gerontology, 62(2), 226-237.

[15] Robinson, L., Hutchings, D., Corner, L., Finch, J., Hughes, J., Brittain, K., et al. (2007). Balancing rights and risks: Conflicting perspectives in the management of wandering in dementia. Health, Risk & Society, 9, 389-406.

[16] Schulz, R., Wahl, H. W., Matthews, J. T., De Vito Dabbs, A., Beach, S. R., & Czaja, S. J. (2015). Advancing the aging and technology agenda in gerontology. The Gerontologist, 55(5), 724-734.

[17] Superflux. 2015. Uninvited guests. Video. 2015. Retrieved May 15, 2019 from https://vimeo.com/172893044.

[18] Vermeer, Y., Higgs, P., & Charlesworth, G. (2019). What do we require from surveillance technology? A review of the needs of people with dementia and informal caregivers. Journal of Rehabilitation and Assistive Technologies Engineering, 6, 2055668319869517.

[19] Walsham, G. (2006). Doing interpretive research. European journal of information systems, 15(3), 320-330.

Healthier Lives, Digitally Enabled
M. Merolli et al. (Eds.)
© 2021 The authors and IOS Press.
This article is published online with Open Access by IOS Press and distributed under the terms
of the Creative Commons Attribution Non-Commercial License 4.0 (CC BY-NC 4.0).
doi:10.3233/SHTI210004

Insights from Public Health Researchers into the Digital Transformation of an Educational Lifestyle Course

William BEVENS [a], Kathleen GRAY [a], Tracey WEILAND [a] and George JELINEK [a]
[a] The University of Melbourne, IOS Press, Australia

Abstract. The last decade has seen an explosion in the uptake of digital health interventions (DHI) to address complex chronic diseases. This is particularly true in the case of multiple sclerosis where those living with the disease are increasingly seeking adjuvant treatment options such as lifestyle management. This paper seeks to give perspectives and insights from public health researchers that have engaged in the digital transformation process of a face-to-face lifestyle management educational program. There is a dearth of information regarding the digital transformation of lifestyle educational programs and this is particularly true for programs directed at chronic diseases. A large body of work exists from higher education, an area that has undergone rapid digital transformation of its work, and much can be derived from this field. There is also a well-established field of design methodologies and frameworks available to researchers seeking to design, develop and implement DHIs. This paper provides a practical overview of the synthesis between digital transformation processes in higher education and the application of an existing development framework for DHIs. By describing this process, we hope to fill an existing gap within the literature that will provide a valuable tool for future researchers.

Keywords. digital health interventions, digital transformation, chronic disease, lifestyle education

1. Introduction

Multiple sclerosis (MS) is a chronic, degenerative, autoimmune disease that affects the central nervous system in around 2.3 million people worldwide. The disease course of MS is highly variable (1); the prognosis for those newly diagnosed provides little certainty in how significantly and rapidly the disease may progress. As there is no cure currently available, treating the underlying disease course as well as the associated perturbations is an important concept for MS. There now exists a large body of evidence implicating the role of environmental and lifestyle factors into the health outcomes for people with MS (PwMS) (2, 3). These factors include diet, exercise, smoking, vitamin D and sun exposure and stress. Ultimately, the strong epidemiological basis for some of these factors have yet to be translated into gold standard randomised control trial data, particularly not in combination. This prevents mainstream acceptance of tailored lifestyle recommendations and therefore future research should focus its efforts on high-quality randomised control trials (RCTs) in order to traverse this gap.

The most comprehensive evidence for a multimodal lifestyle intervention comes from the STOP-MS study run by our team. This longitudinal study tracks a large cohort of PwMS that have undertaken a 5-day in-person live-in education program aimed at educating participants on the Overcoming Multiple Sclerosis (OMS) 7-step program that provides best-practice information on diet, physical activity, smoking cessation, vitamin D and stress reduction. Results from this longitudinal study have spanned 5 years of follow-up, showing an improvement and sustainment of a range of important health outcomes for PwMS (4-6). However, significant limitations impede the conducting of RCTs testing face-to-face multimodal lifestyle interventions, which include prohibitive costs, accessibility concerns, maintenance of behavioural change and recruitment, including issues around randomisation and blinding.

Through the use of digital health technologies, many of these limitations can be overcome. Therefore, our team is undertaking the digital transformation of the existing face-to-face OMS lifestyle educational course into a web-based format. Currently, while there are a number of valuable resources for researchers to develop DHIs, they often lack the generalisability required for public health researchers generally and specifically, for the digital transformation process required for our purposes. Further, the process of translating a pre-existing face-to-face course aimed at behavioural change is not a process that is well described in the literature and research teams themselves are often not experienced or lack the skills to appropriately apply these resources. There are key considerations that are not present when designing DHIs without prior material and therefore this needs to be explored further.

This paper will provide insights into the digital transformation process for behavioural change interventions with particular emphasis on the experiences of public health researchers. Due to the increasing utilisation of DHIs and the dearth of information regarding a digital transformation process, we believe it necessary to communicate our experiences and insights into this design and development process, which this paper seeks to do.

2. Design Methodologies

Despite the wealth of information available to researchers to aid in the design stages of DHIs with many groups having advanced their own models or theories to aid in a methodological approach to development, these remain underutilised by research teams developing DHIs outside the health informatics space. In a recent unpublished review on DHIs for PwMS, we found that only 6 out of 17 studies included reported any description of a process design or methodology in the development of their intervention. While often it is difficult to ascertain whether there exists a genuine lack of the use of any framework or whether it is a lack of reporting, authors were surveyed who confirmed these data. Significantly, this made it difficult to replicate previous methods that showed success in these studies, which is a problem more broadly for DHIs (7). This poses an important question: what is required to fill this gap between the established field of DHI design methodologies and the explosion in utilisation of DHIs to address health issues?

2.1. Research Silos

In our experience, this problem relates to an issue of 'research siloing' whereby the skills of an entire discipline, that being digital health and health informatics, were not present within our research group. This is likely to be the case in most public health research groups and is definitely the case within our department and school. In particular, public health informatics research is not highly visible in Australia (8), and this requires researchers to make connections into discplines previously unexplored. In our case, this was straightforward due to working within a large, well-resourced institution, with a School of Computing and Information Systems, E-research group and vast array of online resources. This may not be the case for many other institutions and therefore should be considered an important part of any institution's future plans. Overall, while the idea of interdisciplinary collaboration is not novel, the value of a contemporary discipline such as health informatics needs to be appreciated by more traditional disciplines such as public health.

This may be explained by the attitudes towards digital health by health researchers themselves. Academics may be perceived as lacking technological skills, which may translate to their dismissal of its overall value in academia (9). Further, cost-effectiveness, rather than effectiveness on the health outcomes of interest has been described as the main driver for adopting digital heath technologies (10), whereby priority is placed on rapid developments at the expense for thorough planning.

Efforts are ongoing to resolve the issue of research 'silos' by recognising the diversity of skills necessary to tackle macro-problems. This is none more evident than in the current effort to tackle the global coronavirus pandemic. Emphasis should be placed on continuing the work in integrating health informatics within disciplines, including public health.

3. Digital Transformation

There is likely to be a difference in approach required between a digital transformation project such as ours, and a project whereby a DHI is designed from scratch. This is an unexplored area within the literature; while there exist interventions that have been 'digitised', the experiences taken from this process or the underlying methodology have not been well-reported. It is clear that many existing interventions will undergo a digitisation in the future and therefore, explorations of this process are vital.

For the purposes of our project, this transformation process involved augmenting the initial stages of the design process. As is recognised across the majority of digital health development frameworks, the initial stages of this process are to be characterised by analysis of the needs of end-users and the context in which the intervention will be implemented. For our purposes, the framework we selected was the CeHReS roadmap (11) due to its amalgamation of participatory design and persuasive design elements, described in a way that was understandable to our research team.

For a digital transformation project, this initial step will vary slightly in its intended use because the problem statement is likely already identified. Further. that intervention may have already undergone extensive quantitative and qualitative testing to uncover both the mechanism of action of participant experiences with the intervention. This was the case with our intervention as we had more than a decade of delivery to many hundreds of PwMS and multiple quantitative and qualitative publications. One example is that our research team already recognised the necessity of accessibility features due to potential for participants within our cohort to present with physical and/or cognitive impairments. What remained for us in terms of a digital transformation process was to understand the problems associated with the current format of delivery, the solutions that may emerge from a digital platform and to address the limitations associated with this transformation.

3.1. Advisory Group

This process took place utilising an advisory group of PwMS from the community. This group comprised those who had previous experience with the face-to-face program and other associated resources whilst others had heard of the program but had very little exposure to it. This group, through semi-structured group conversations, provided insight into a wide range of important aspects of the pre-existing course and elements that should be considered for a digital course. In particular, two important elements of the existing course were identified from these discussions as areas to which our team should pay close attention: peer support and experts delivering content. It was recognised that the transformation of these two key elements into a digital environment was a key aspect to the success of this project. The process of elucidating key components of a pre-existing behavioural change intervention by both the research team and end-users via the contextual inquiry stage of design facilitates this process.

These two themes were then interrogated as to how they exerted their intended effect on the outcome of interest in the existing course, and then how they may operate within the digital space. In terms of our project, this meant exploring what was successful about the experts delivering educational content and the peer-support elements of the course, which in turn drove behavioural changes that led to improved health previously described.

3.2. Expert Educational Content

Formal educational content process within the face-to-face course was delivered via seminar style presentations led by experts (physicians, researchers or dieticians) in their chosen discipline. Briefly, these seminars covered topics on diet, physical activity, stress reduction, sun exposure and vitamin D, medication and family prevention. The format of these seminars followed an informal structure of 'why' and 'how': firstly, clinical and research data was presented on a topic and illustrated visually with figures and images; secondly, information was provided on how to implement the recommendations according to the research data previously presented.

The practical, physical task of transforming the content will occur between researchers and developers, be they researchers as well or industry professionals. For our purposes, once the types and frequency of multimedia elements to exist in the platform was decided, content templates were generated by the development team, and these templates were then filled by members of the research team. This methodical approach of content implementation was a skill our research team was not familiar with and one that was introduced by the industry professional team.

3.3. Peer-support

The benefits of peer-support for chronic diseases within digital environments has been previously described and contain a range of synchronous and asynchronous approaches (12). The benefits and limitations of any particular approach needed to be considered by the research team. In our case, these benefits and negatives were informed both on our prior experiences with the face-to-face course and the opinions raised within the advisory group. In the face-to-face course, participants would learn from others in an experiential, peer-support manner, which was unstructured and could occur any time participants interacted. It is important to note that because the face-to-face course is a 5-day residential course, interaction occurs consistently as participants go about their daily activities. This is not feasible in a modular, online educational course and therefore useful alternatives needed to be considered.

The advisory group was split on the implementation of a synchronous chat system but ultimately agreed that there were alternatives outside the platform that may be preferable. The "anonymity" of a DHI would give participants pause to use a synchronous tool to communicate with each other due to the perceived inability to develop emotional connections in the online course format. Participants indicated that they had prior experience engaging with forums, particularly those familiar with OMS program who had engaged with the OMS forums, and that would be a comfortable medium for peer-to-peer interaction for an online course.

With this information, it was decided that the peer-support component (experiential content) would be facilitated using an asynchronous forum system with light moderation. This method of peer-support is a large deviation from how this occurs within the face-to-face program for three important reasons: it occurs in a virtual space as opposed to physical; it is asynchronous; and participants are aware of moderation and that their communication is visible to the wider groups. It is not clear what the outcomes of these differences will be however future feasibility testing will clarify this.

3.4. Development Team

Choosing a development team is a difficult decision, as the majority of researchers will lack the understanding of the skills and expertise required to undertake a project as large and important as many DHIs. Additionally, while the field of DHIs is relatively new as an academic discipline, it is novel as a venture for small businesses also, who may seek to enter into this market with little experience in this field. For all these reasons, our team initially found ourselves engaged with a contractor that was unable to deliver upon our intended design. It is unclear how common this is as the design and development process is often not articulated fully and appropriately within the literature. Fortunately, through a series of networking processes, we located a team who had previously interacted with the facilitators of the residential course and with the general skills and experience to engage in a task such as ours. Interdisciplinary collaboration will give research teams the resources and skills to both find, vet and collaborate with development teams.

4. Summary

Based upon the issues and insights raised in this paper, we propose some key recommendations for research teams and institutions:

1. *Ensuring research groups are multidisciplinary.* An appreciation of the complexity involved in the design, development and administering of DHIs is required by public health researchers, which will ideally lead to the incorporation of health informatics researchers into their groups.
2. *Provide centralised lists of recommended developers.* This is critical in ensuring that researchers are engaging those that are best equipped to develop DHIs alongside researchers. As it is often difficult for researchers with little knowledge of DHIs to recognise what skills are needed, a list such as this would be invaluable.
3. *The development of digital transformation methodologies.* Much of this process can be informed from existing design methodologies and frameworks dedicated

to digital health however, there remain elements specific to transformational projects that are unaccounted for in these models.

Ultimately, we believe implementing these key recommendations will allow researchers greater access to better resources that will ensure DHIs are appropriately designed, developed and therefore, adequately evaluated.

References

[1]   Tsang BK, Macdonell R. Multiple sclerosis- diagnosis, management and prognosis. Australian family physician. 2011;40(12):948-55.

[2]   Jakimovski D, Guan Y, Ramanathan M, Weinstock-Guttman B, Zivadinov R. Lifestyle-based modifiable risk factors in multiple sclerosis: review of experimental and clinical findings. Neurodegener Dis Manag. 2019;9(3):149-72.

[3]   Belbasis L, Bellou V, Evangelou E, Ioannidis JP, Tzoulaki I. Environmental risk factors and multiple sclerosis: an umbrella review of systematic reviews and meta-analyses. Lancet Neurol. 2015;14(3):263-73.

[4]   Hadgkiss EJ, Jelinek GA, Weiland TJ, Rumbold G, Mackinlay CA, Gutbrod S, et al. Health-related quality of life outcomes at 1 and 5 years after a residential retreat promoting lifestyle modification for people with multiple sclerosis. Neurol Sci. 2013;34(2):187-95.

[5]   Li MP, Jelinek GA, Weiland TJ, Mackinlay CA, Dye S, Gawler I. Effect of a residential retreat promoting lifestyle modifications on health-related quality of life in people with multiple sclerosis. Quality in primary care. 2010;18(6):379-89.

[6]   Marck CH, De Livera AM, Brown CR, Neate SL, Taylor KL, Weiland TJ, et al. Health outcomes and adherence to a healthy lifestyle after a multimodal intervention in people with multiple sclerosis: Three year follow-up. PLoS One. 2018;13(5):e0197759.

[7]   Coiera E, Ammenwerth E, Georgiou A, Magrabi F. Does health informatics have a replication crisis? Journal of the American Medical Informatics Association. 2018;25(8):963-8.

[8]   Gray K, Martin Sanchez F. Public Health Informatics in Australia and around the World. Public Health Informatics in Australia and around the World. Telehealth and Mobile Health: Taylor; 2015.

[9]   Sucala M, Nilsen W, Muench F. Building partnerships: a pilot study of stakeholders' attitudes on technology disruption in behavioral health delivery and research. Translational Behavioral Medicine. 2017;7(4):854-60.

[10]   Topooco N, Riper H, Araya R, Berking M, Brunn M, Chevreul K, et al. Attitudes towards digital treatment for depression: A European stakeholder survey. Internet Interventions. 2017;8:1-9.

[11]   van Gemert-Pijnen JE, Nijland N, van Limburg M, Ossebaard HC, Kelders SM, Eysenbach G, et al. A Holistic Framework to Improve the Uptake and Impact of eHealth Technologies. J Med Internet Res. 2011;13(4):e111.

[12]   Merolli M, Gray K, Martin Sanchez F. Health outcomes and related effects of using social media in chronic disease management: a literature review and analysis of affordances. J Biomed Inform. 2013;46(6):957-69.

Healthier Lives, Digitally Enabled
M. Merolli et al. (Eds.)
© *2021 The authors and IOS Press.*
This article is published online with Open Access by IOS Press and distributed under the terms
of the Creative Commons Attribution Non-Commercial License 4.0 (CC BY-NC 4.0).
doi:10.3233/SHTI210005

Towards Automatic and Interpretable Assignments of Patients Presenting with Pain to the Emergency Department

JA HUGHES [a,b,1], NJ BROWN [a,c], Thanh VU [d] and Anthony NGUYEN [d]

[a] *Emergency and Trauma Centre, Royal Brisbane and Women's Hospital, Brisbane, Australia*
[b] *School of Nursing, Queensland University of Technology, Brisbane, Australia*
[c] *Faculty of Medicine, University of Queensland, Brisbane, Australia*
[d] *Australian e-Health Research Centre, CSIRO, Brisbane, Australia*

Introduction. Pain is the most common symptom that patients present with to the emergency department. It is hard to identify patients who have presented in pain to the emergency department when compliance with structured pain assessment is low. An ability to identify patients presenting in pain allows further investigation of the quality of care provided. **Background.** Machine and deep learning techniques are commonly used for text analysis in healthcare. Applications such as the classification of diagnosis and unplanned readmissions from textual medical records have previously been described. In other work, conventional and deep-learning techniques have demonstrated high performance in identifying patients presenting to the emergency department in pain. However, these models have lacked interpretability. **Methods.** This paper proposes the use of machine learning techniques to identify patients who present in pain based upon their initial assessment using interpretable deep learning models. **Results.** The interpretable deep learning model of pain identification was shown to have more accuracy and precision than other machine and deep learning techniques. This technique has significant application to large datasets for the identification of the quality of care and real-time identification of patients presenting in pain to improve their care.

Keywords. pain, Emergency Department, machine learning, deep learning, nursing assessment

1. Introduction

Pain is the most common symptom that patients experience when they present to the emergency department (ED) [1], with between 65% [2] and 78% [3] of all presentations experiencing pain. In the ED, pain assessment and treatment have been reported as poor, leading to increased wait times and unnecessary symptom burden and suffering [4; 5]. Identification of patients who present with pain has long been a pillar of pain care in the ED but is poorly completed. Pain is a subjective experience and is best described and identified by the person experiencing it [6]. Clinical staff have previously been shown to be poor predictors of the presence and severity of pain [7; 8], with the patient's self-

---

[1] Corresponding Author, Dr James Hughes, Emergency and Trauma Centre, Royal Brisbane and Women's Hospital, Butterfield Street Herston; E-mail: james.hughes@health.qld.gov.au.

report of pain the most reliable indicator. In the absence of documented pain assessment, identifying patients who may have presented in pain can be difficult, and therefore alternative methods for identifying patients in pain are needed for; identifying prevalence of pain on presentation, assessing the outcomes of quality improvement activities and for use in real time to prompt clinicians to assess and treat patients presenting in pain. Others have previously described a method of manually identifying patients in pain using free text triage nursing assessments [9] that is not reliant on severity scoring, however this methodology at a large scale would be time consuming, laborious and impractical.

Machine learning is widely used in healthcare for predictive tasks such as, cancer staging from pathology reports [10], diagnosis from medical records [11; 12], and mortality and unplanned readmissions [13]. The increasing availability of large datasets collected by electronic medical records allows machine learning to be used to improve the quality of care provided to patients [10-12; 14]. To overcome the limitations of manual identification, Vu et al. [20] proposed to use machine learning including both conventional and deep learning models [15-19] to learn patterns in text that identify patients presenting with pain to the ED. Although the proposed machine learning models achieved high performances on the task, they were "black boxes" and do not explain *"how the model makes its decisions,"* which is a fundamental question in healthcare analytics. This paper proposes a interpretable deep learning model to handle the problem.

2. Methods

This study aims to formally introduce and test a method of identification of patients presenting to the ED in pain using conventional machine learning and deep learning techniques. To achieve this aim, it is herein described the construction of a dataset of ED patients from a large inner-city adult ED to evaluate the proposed machine learning models. In these models, each patient is assigned as either "Pain" denoting they presented with pain or "No Pain" denoting they arrived without pain as a presenting symptom.

2.1. Task Description

The task described in this work is a binary description of the presence of pain on arrival to the ED, either the patient has "Pain" or "No Pain". To achieve this task, unstructured free text of the nursing assessment and presenting problem entered into the electronic medical record at triage is used. Table 1 demonstrates examples of the unstructured free text that indicated both the presence of "Pain" and "No Pain". As can be seen, by these examples, the task is complicated by shorthand notation, abbreviations and typographical errors.

Table 1. Examples of unstructured free-text from the presenting problem and nursing assessment fields of the electronic medical record. Highlighted terms are indicative of pain.

"Presenting Problem" and "Nursing Assessment"	Class
2/24 frontal headache/ photophobia/ lower l) back urinary incontinence	"Pain"
? Seizure activity// not on meds// elevated post drug use hx of drug use	"No Pain"

2.2. Dataset

The ED data manager extracted the dataset comprised of a random selection of 2000 patients presenting to an inner-city Australian ED between August and October 2018. A medical student under the supervision of a senior clinician/researcher assigned each patient either a "Pain" or "No Pain" label based on the information contained in the presenting problem and nursing assessment free text fields. The student searched the free text for keywords indicating pain, or for a pain intensity assessment ("xx/10") or descriptor ("mild pain"), and assigned a "Pain" or "No Pain" label to each case accordingly. This dataset was then split into three datasets (Training, Development and Test) as per Table 2 below.

Table 2. Basic Dataset Statistics

Dataset	Patients	Pain	No-Pain
Training	1200	574 (48%)	626 (52%)
Development	400	171 (43%)	229 (57%)
Test	400	193 (48%)	207 (52%)
Total	2000	938 (47%)	1062 (53%)

2.3. Interpretable Deep Learning Model

The interpretable deep learning model builds upon performant artificial recurrent neural networks (RNN) applied on the same dataset [20]. In contrast to Vu et al. [20], an attention layer is added to help the model attend to important information (i.e., input words). The attention weights given by the layer for each input word can be used to help explain what the model did to produce the output label. In particular, more important words contributing to a label would be associated with higher attention weights. Figure 1 illustrates our AttRNN model architecture.

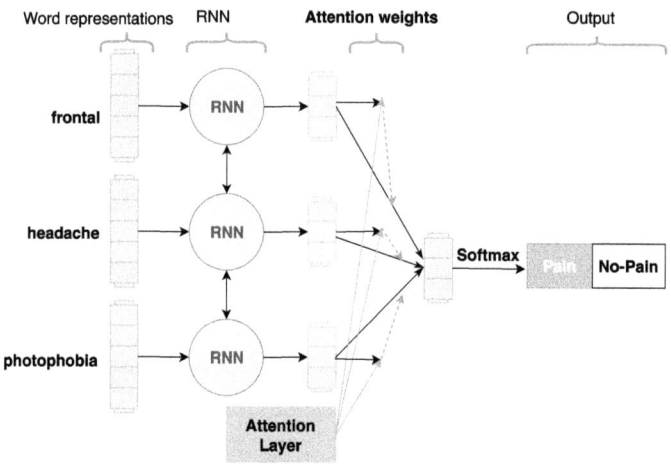

Figure 1. Attention-based Recurrent Neural Network model architecture (AttRNN)

The input to the model consists of a vector representation of words from the electronic medical record of a patient. The vector representations were learnt in advance on a large-scale clinical dataset using a word representation model. *RNN* takes the vector representation of each word and produces an output vector for that word. The attention layer produces *attention weights* for each word. The final vector was generated using the *RNN* output vectors and the attention weights. The final vector was then used to predict the class of the input record (i.e., either "Pain" or "No-Pain") as the output of the model. In Figure 1, the model classifies a "Pain" label for the "… frontal headache photophobia …" input text. The model was learnt and finetuned on the Training and Development set, respectively. The model effectiveness will be reported on the unseen Test set.

3. Results

The performance of the interpretable deep learning model, AttRNN, was compared with other models proposed by Vu et al. [20], RULE - a rule-based model, Support Vector Machine (SVM) - a conventional machine learning model and Recurrent Neural Network (RNN) – a deep learning model. Table 3 shows the experimental results of the models on the test set. Note that AttRNN is an extension of RNN with an additional attention layer which helps explain the model output. In particular, we can see that the results produced by AttRNN are competitive with the state-of-the-art results produced by RNN, a deep learning model. More importantly, the produced attention weights of AttRNN can be used to visualise the importance of each word within the input text making the model interpretable. Table 4 shows examples of using attention weights produced by AttRNN to help interpret the results. In particular, *"headache photophobia"* and *"pain behind l ear"* are highlighted as more relevant to the "pain" label. It is worth noting that this interpretability feature is not available with RNN.

Table 3. Experimental results (%) on the test set. ∗ indicates that the performance difference between the machine learning models and the RULE model is significant at the significance level α of 0.1 using the Approximate Randomisation test [3, 5]. + indicates that the results are taken from Vu et al. [20].

| Model | Accuracy (%) | Macro-averaged | | |
		Precision (%)	Recall (%)	F_1 (%)
RULE+	84.75	84.87	84.63	84.69
SVM+	88.00	88.13*	87.90*	87.96*
RNN+	**91.00***	91.21*	**90.88***	**90.96***
AttRNN	**91.00***	91.43*	90.83*	90.94*

Table 4. AttRNN generated attention weights for interpreting the output.

Output	Input Interpretation
Pain	2 24 frontal headache photophobia lower l back urinary incontinence
Pain	Aloc and seizure activity post 2 unit blood donation today pain behind l ear

4. Discussion

The immediate application of the research is to provide interpretable machine learning assistance to identify patients presenting in pain over a very large, statewide dataset. This will allow the authors to answer the initial question of pain prevalence on presentation to the ED in Queensland and lead to the ability to explore the assessment and treatment of pain over a large population. Future applications include the potential real-time clinical application, such as a smart support assistant to help improve the quality of triage related to presentations that involve or are likely to involve pain. The gold standard in pain care is still universal assessment, clinicians at the bedside must assess and document a patient's pain. Tools such as the one described in this work will hopefully assist this in the longer term.

This paper proposed an interpretable deep learning model for the task of identifying patients who presented to EDs with pain. Experimental results on a 2,000 ED patient annotated dataset showed that not only this model performed well on this task with the highest accuracy and macro-averaged F_1 score of 91.00% and 90.94%, respectively, which are similar to the state-of-the-art results from a RNN [20], but also attention weights can be further used for visualisation making the model output interpretable which is the important and unique feature of the proposed model.

These learnings are beneficial for similar text classification research on other clinical tasks, such as cancer staging from pathology reports [10], diagnosis coding from medical records [11; 12], and prediction of mortality and unplanned readmissions [13]. It also sets a solid foundation for further improving performances on the "pain" models to scale the "pain" study to other hospitals and regions.

References

[1]   K.H. Todd, A review of current and emerging approaches to pain management in the emergency department, *J Pain Therapy* **6** (2017), 193-202.
[2]   Care Quality Commission., 2016 Emergency Department Survey: Statistical Release, in: Q.C. Commission, ed., National Health Service, London, 2016.
[3]   F. Karwowski-Soulié, S. Lessenot-Tcherny, A. Lamarche-Vadel, S. Bineau, C. Ginsburg, O. Meyniard, B. Mendoza, P. Fodella, G. Vidal-Trecan, and F. Brunet, Pain in an emergency department: an audit, *European Journal of Emergency Medicine* **13** (2006), 218-224.
[4]   W. Varndell, M. Fry, and D. Elliott, Quality and impact of nurse-initiated analgesia in the emergency department: A systematic review, *International emergency nursing* **40** (2018), 46-53.
[5]   C. Hatherley, N. Jennings, and R. Cross, Time to analgesia and pain score documentation best practice standards for the emergency department–a literature review, *Australasian Emergency Nursing Journal* **19** (2016), 26-36.
[6]   A.C. Williams and K.D. Craig, Updating the definition of pain, *J Pain* **157** (2016), 2420-2423.
[7]   L. Marquié, E. Raufaste, D. Lauque, C. Mariné, M. Ecoiffier, and P. Sorum, Pain rating by patients and physicians: evidence of systematic pain miscalibration, *Journal of Pain* **102** (2003), 289-296.
[8]   M. Duignan and V. Dunn, Congruence of pain assessment between nurses and emergency department patients: a replication, *International emergency nursing* **16** (2008), 23-28.
[9]   J.A. Hughes, N.J. Brown, J. Chiu, B. Allwood, and K. Chu, The relationship between time to analgesic administration and emergency department length of stay: A retrospective review, *Journal of Advanced Nursing* (2019).
[10] I. McCowan, D. Moore, and M.-J. Fry, Classification of cancer stage from free-text histology reports, in: *2006 International Conference of the IEEE Engineering in Medicine and Biology Society*, IEEE, 2006, pp. 5153-5156.
[11] B. Koopman, G. Zuccon, A. Nguyen, A. Bergheim, and N. Grayson, Automatic ICD-10 classification of cancers from free-text death certificates, *International journal of medical informatics* **84** (2015), 956-965.

[12] J. Mullenbach, S. Wiegreffe, J. Duke, J. Sun, and J. Eisenstein, Explainable prediction of medical codes from clinical text, *Proceedings of the 2018 Conference of the North American Chapter* (2018).

[13] A. Rajkomar, E. Oren, K. Chen, A.M. Dai, N. Hajaj, M. Hardt, P.J. Liu, X. Liu, J. Marcus, and M. Sun, Scalable and accurate deep learning with electronic health records, *Digital Medicine* **1** (2018), 18.

[14] Z. Che, J.S. Sauver, H. Liu, and Y. Liu, Deep learning solutions for classifying patients on opioid use, in: *AMIA Annual Symposium Proceedings*, American Medical Informatics Association, 2017, p. 525.

[15] B. Scholkopf and A.J. Smola, Learning with kernels: support vector machines, regularization, optimization, and beyond, MIT press, 2001.

[16] A. Liaw and M. Wiener, Classification and regression by Random Forest, *R News* **2** (2002), 18-22.

[17] J.L. Elman, Finding structure in time, *Cognitive science* **14** (1990), 179-211.

[18] Y. LeCun, L. Bottou, Y. Bengio, and P. Haffner, Gradient-based learning applied to document recognition, *Proceedings of the IEEE* **86** (1998), 2278-2324.

[19] J. Chung, C. Gulcehre, K. Cho, and Y. Bengio, Empirical evaluation of gated recurrent neural networks on sequence modeling, *NIPS 2014 Workshop on Deep Learning* (2014).

[20] T. Vu, A. Nguyen, N. Brown, and J. Hughes, Identifying patients with pain in emergency departments using conventional machine learning and deep learning, in: *Proceedings of the The 17th Annual Workshop of the Australasian Language Technology Association*, 2019, pp. 111-119.

Healthier Lives, Digitally Enabled
M. Merolli et al. (Eds.)
© 2021 The authors and IOS Press.
This article is published online with Open Access by IOS Press and distributed under the terms
of the Creative Commons Attribution Non-Commercial License 4.0 (CC BY-NC 4.0).
doi:10.3233/SHTI210006

Pandora's Bot: Insights from the Syntax and Semantics of Suicide Notes

David IRELAND [a,1] and DanaKai BRADFORD [a]

[a] Australian e-Health Research Centre, CSIRO

Abstract. Conversation agents (chat-bots) are becoming ubiquitous in many domains of everyday life, including physical and mental health and wellbeing. With the high rate of suicide in Australia, chat-bot developers are facing the challenge of dealing with statements related to mental ill-health, depression and suicide. Advancements in natural language processing could allow for sensitive, considered responses, provided suicidal discourse can be accurately detected. Here suicide notes are examined for consistent linguistic syntax and semantic patterns used by individuals in mental health distress. *Paper contains distressing content.*

Keywords. natural language processing, chat-bots, suicide, mental health

1. Introduction

In Greek mythology, Pandora was given a box of 'gifts', which upon opening released grief and woe into the world. As she hurriedly closed the box, one gift was trapped within – Hope [1]. This parallels the world in which people contemplating suicide live, where there is much suffering and despair, while aspiration seems unattainable.

Suicide is the leading cause of the death for individuals aged between 15-44 in Australia and has a per-capita rate of 12.1% as of 2018 [2,3]. The most significant risk factor for death by suicide is a history of mental illness [3]. This may be further exacerbated by stigmatisation, resulting in a 'wall of silence' around suicide, supported by avoidance, denial and dismissive community and/or family attitudes [4], that makes it difficult for people with suicide ideation to verbalise their experience and seek help.

Conversation agents (also known as chat-bots) are undergoing an exponential growth in development, with applications for a range of supporting roles, from virtual assistants such as Apple's Siri and Amazon's Alexa, to therapy aids for Parkinson's disease, Autism Spectrum Disorder, genetic counselling and mental health [5-11]. Recent advancements in automatic speech recognition have been a catalyst for computer programs processing and responding to natural language. There is, however, the potential for negative consequences, such as privacy and ethical violations.

A fascinating aspect of language, and hence challenge for natural language processing, is that grammar allows for the construction of sentences that have never been uttered [12]. It is therefore conceivable that chat-bot users will convey statements that were not expected by the original developers. An historic example of this is early versions of Siri which responded to the phrase "*I want to jump off a bridge and die*" by giving directions to the nearest bridge [13]. This was quickly rectified, and Siri's

---

[1] Corresponding Author

responses are now more appropriate [14]. None-the-less, this exemplifies why statements related to mental health need significant consideration; both ethically, and legally if developers will be held accountable for the chat-bot responses.

With the ubiquitous presence of chat-bots, there is an open question as to what role these agents will play in more complex human affairs and how they will be developed. Here we propose the use of suicide notes to develop a skeleton framework for detecting utterances indicative of suicide ideation, or poor mental health and wellbeing. Suicide notes are often the last articulated expression of sentiment before the individual acts to take their life. A Queensland study found that a written note accompanied 39% of suicides in 2004 [15], and in general, note leavers tend to be socio-demographically representative of the wider suicide population [15,16]. Whilst it is acknowledged they are often precious mementos to the families; these notes offer forms of communication with invaluable insight into the reasoning processes stated by the individual and the language syntax and semantic styles used to convey their state of mind at the time of writing.

While negative dialogue for melancholy, despair and sadness can be easily emulated, there is evidence that natural language processing algorithms can more accurately distinguish genuine from simulated suicide notes than a human expert [17]. Thus, it is argued there are inherent linguistic patterns and cognitive styles that could contribute to a body of knowledge around suicidal discourse. Moreover, it is likely that the linguistic and cognitive patterns detected in a corpus of suicide notes would manifest earlier in individuals with suicide ideation and general mental health distress.

This paper briefly describes the origin and demographics of the suicide notes used and the chat-bot framework into which they were incorporated. We then explore the characteristic language patterns of suicidal discourse that require novel language processing algorithms. It is not our intention to develop a 'suicide prevention chat-bot' per se, but rather to understand how to detect suicide-related syntax and semantics in any chat-bot interaction. Developing appropriate responses, together with qualified professionals, is a challenge for another day. Finally, we provide our own last thoughts.

2. Leaving Last Words - Suicide Note Data Set

Use of the following corpus of written suicide notes was approved by the CSIRO Health and Medical Human Research Ethics Committee (178/19). The first set comprises notes written by males (n=33) aged 25-29 during the years 1945-54 [18]. The second set includes notes written by males (n=32) and females (n=20) aged 25-29 during 1983-84. Both sets were originally sourced from the Coroner's Office at Los Angeles County, California, United States [19]. To increase diversity and recency, we conducted an internet search and collated a third set from publicly available notes, written by males (n=4), females (n=6) and a transgender female, aged 14-85 spanning 1932-2019, from across the world. For privacy, quotes are attributed only by gender and year. Most of the notes indicate psychological pain, and 10, including the eldest three (aged 67-85, one female) suffered significant physical pain in the years preceding their suicide. All 96 authors ended their lives.

3. Chat-Bot Framework

The chat-bot framework is an in-house development project [7,8], with input via speech or text. It has a case-based reasoner and a logic reasoner that operate on the syntax and semantics of the human utterance respectively.

The case-based reasoner is the main workhorse of the chat-bot and provides most of the responses and the virtual personality of the chat-bot. It uses two main algorithms [8,20], a syntactic matching algorithm and a sentiment analysis algorithm that supports the case-based reasoner by alerting the chat-bot when negative sentiment has been uttered. Our chat-bot can be encoded with multiple responses, with each specific response chosen based on the sentiment of the last utterance and overall conversation.

The logic reasoner acts on the computed semantics of the human utterance. Wordnet, a large lexicon database consisting of word types, synonyms and antonyms [21], is used to support the logic reasoner in converting natural language to the language of logic. This allows representation of natural language data, detection of logical contradictions, and response to queries that can be resolved logically.

4. Characteristic Language Patterns of Suicidal Discourse

The transformation of the suicide notes into the chat-bot framework took into account four main language patterns. The first two are derived from Shneidman's theory [18, 22,23] which postulates that suicidal ideations are often characterised by constrictive thinking and logical fallacies. These patterns have been empirically validated [19]. We further found that language idioms and negative sentiment were also idiosyncratic.

4.1. Constrictive Thinking - "...I will never escape the darkness or misery..." (M, 2011)

Constrictive thinking only considers the absolute when dealing with a protracted source of distress, there is no compromise. The language of constrictive thinking contains terms such as *either/or, always, never, forever, nothing, totally, all* and *only* - terms typically found in the adverbial phrase of the grammar constituent (Suicide Quote 1). All identified constrictive terms were encoded in the case-based reasoner and included in the sentiment analyser.

*"I'm sorry it seems **the only way**."* (M, 1983-4)

Suicide Quote 1. An example of a sentence containing constrictive language (bold, underlined).

4.2. Logical Fallacies - "...Learn from Mistakes, Commit Suicide..." (F, 1983-4)

Illogical reasoning often manifests in the suicide note. Frequently, the author is expressing a set premise as to why they are taking this course of action. General logical contradictions and fallacies are of interest, but the most common type of fallacy is called catastrophic logic or catalogic (as it leads to the catastrophic cessation of the reasoner) [22,23]. A core characteristic of catalogic is semantic fallacy (Suicide Quote 2). In this example, the semantic fallacy relates to the meaning of the pronoun *I*, the definition of which changes between the two clauses that make up the second sentence. This fallacy occurs when the author expresses that they will experience feelings such as happiness or success after their own death. It has been postulated this pattern occurs when the individual cannot imagine their own death [18,23].

"I am tired of failing. ***If I can do this I will succeed.****"* (M, 1983-4)

Suicide Quote 2. An example of a semantic fallacy (bold, underlined) common in the suicide note dataset.

The detection of this fallacy is technically challenging and goes beyond classical logic programming as numerous paradoxes emerge when transforming natural language statements that deal with implications into a formal system [24,25]. Our approach is experimental and utilises a dynamic deontic logic system [25] that considers actions (verbs) and states (adjectives) as unique domains. Special notation is used to represent a consequent state φ after action α is performed as $[\alpha](\varphi)$. The logical representation of Suicide Note 2 derived by our chat-bot logic reasoner is given in Eq (1) where the action '*this*' has been anaphorically referenced (from content earlier in the interaction) to mean the suicide act. The user of the chat-bot is denoted by x; $\wedge$ indicates the conjunction operator, and the special operators indicate the action $[\alpha]$ [in this case, suicide] and the consequent state (φ) (in this case, success).

$$Tired\ (x,\ failure)\ \wedge\ [suicide(x)]\ (success(x)) \tag{1}$$

The semantic fallacy here is that entity x will not exist after the act of suicide thus the consequent state will not occur. To counter this, our chat-bot has pre-encoded axioms in the same vein as Asimov's Three Laws of Robotics [26]. Eq (2) gives an example axiom that would contradict the statement given in Eq (1) and alert the chat-bot. The method of analytic tableaux (a decision tree for logical formula) [24] is used to prove the contradiction. In this 2nd order dynamic deontic axiom, $\forall$ denotes the universal all operator and $\neg$ denotes negation. It expresses there are no valid states after entity x has suicided.

$$\forall f\ \forall x\ [suicide(x)]\ (\neg f(x)) \tag{2}$$

4.3. Language Idioms - "The grass is greener on the outher [sic] side" (M, 1983-4)

Language idioms are phrases that chat-bots typically cannot interpret correctly as they are often colloquial, and the meaning of the phrase can be different from the literal meaning (Suicide Quote 3). All found idioms were encoded in the case-based reasoner along with their implied meaning.

"I just checked out. *May God have mercy on my soul."* (M, 1983-4)

Suicide Quote 3. An example of a language idiom (bold, underlined), where a euphemism is used for suicide.

4.4. Negative Sentiment - "... just this heavy, overwhelming despair..." (F, 1983-4)

The majority of notes expressed pervasive negative affect. A sentence was labelled negative sentiment if it referred to any of the following: expressions of dislike or dissatisfaction; melancholy, depression, futility (Suicide Quote 4), sickness, existential crisis, constrictive terms, exhaustion or death; illegal activities; insults and profanity; and communication breakdown or misunderstandings. Statements with negative sentiment were added to the data set of the sentiment analyser in the chat-bot.

"I can't handle the responsibility of life." "This terrible depression keeps coming over me."

Suicide Quote 4. Examples of negative sentiment seen in the majority of notes (both from males in 1983-4).

5. Discussion

We analysed 96 notes penned over nearly 90 years (but predominantly in the 40s and 80s) by authors mainly in their late 20s (90%) but spanning ages 14-85; and identified four main idiosyncratic language patterns including constrictive thinking and illogical reasoning [18,22,23], idioms and negative sentiment. We then programmed these phrases into a chat-bot framework, developing specific algorithms using case-based and logic reasoning, as well as sentiment analysis, to detect these patterns in a chat-bot interaction. Using combined algorithms, the module would detect phrases such as

"I have accepted hope is nothing more than delayed disappointment" (F, 1941).

Interestingly, and perhaps alarmingly, suicide note dialogue seems to have changed little over the last century. There is some evidence that suicide typologies are reflected in suicide note content [28], which raises the question of whether certain groups are more likely to leave notes. However, research suggests there are no socio-demographic differences between people who do and do not leave a note, other than living alone [16]. This study is somewhat contradicted by a recent study in Queensland, which found that the odds of a note being left were slightly lower for females, Aboriginal Australians and those diagnosed with a mental illness [15], although sample sizes in the first two groups were small. An important finding of this second study was that when the definition of 'suicide note' was broadened to include electronic notes and verbal threats, the incidence of 'note' leaving rose to 61%. The likelihood of a handwritten note being left increased with female gender and higher socio-economic status; while being Indigenous or diagnosed with a mental health illness increased the likelihood of a verbal 'note' [15]. Chat-bots, as electronic media with capacity for voice and text, have the potential to capture suicidal discourse from the wider suicide population.

A meta-analysis of over 3000 suicides found that 87% had been diagnosed with a mental disorder [28]. In our dataset, at least 10% of the notes contained reference to physical illness that contributed to a sense of being unable to endure living. The emergence of chat-bots in healthcare for physical and psychological health [e.g. 7,10,11] places this technology in a position to encounter suicidal discourse with perhaps a corresponding responsibility to incorporate a suicide module into the chat-bot development framework.

As chat-bots become increasingly commonplace, so will the user expectations as to the intelligence of the device. While it is possible interactions with chat-bots may be a source of early detection for risk of suicide or mental health distress, there are still the questions of how the chat-bot responds and at what point in time and to whom does the chat-bot alert the need for an intervention. If suicidal thoughts are detected early enough, it is possible that preliminary intervention could be delivered via the chat-bot.

6. Conclusion

Across our dataset, the characteristics of illogical reasoning, constrictive thinking, negative sentiment and idioms were consistent in suicidal discourse. Specific, sensitive and well considered language processing will be required if a suicide module is going to be embedded into chat-bots of the future. If such a module can be developed, then amongst the grief and woe of the suicidal mind, Pandora's bot may just hold *Hope*.

References

[1] https://www.greekmyths-greekmythology.com/pandoras-box-myth/ last accessed 2020-02-10.
[2] Australian Bureau of Statistics, *Causes of Death, Australia, 2018*. Publication no. 3303.0. Canberra.
[3] https://www.suicidepreventionaust.org/wp-content/uploads/2019/11/2019_Sept_SPA_Turning_Points_ White_Paper.pdf
[4] A.L., Calear P.J., Batterham H. Christensen Predictors of help-seeking for suicidal ideation in the community. *Psychiatry Res.* **219**, (2014), 525–530.
[5] Apple Inc., "Siri" https://www.apple.com/au/ios/siri/, last accessed on 2020-02-14.
[6] Amazon.con, Inc., "Amazon Alexa." https://developer.amazon.com/alexa last accessed on 2020-02-14.
[7] D. Ireland, J. Liddle, S. McBride, H. Ding, C. Knuepfer, Chat-Bots for people with Parkinson's Disease: Science Fiction or Reality?, *Studies in Health Technology and Informatics* **214** (2015), 128-33.
[8] D. Ireland, C. Atay, J. Liddle et al. Hello Harlie: Enabling speech monitoring through chat-bot conversations. *Studies in Health Technology and Informatics* **227** (2016), 55-60.
[9] A. Cooper, D. Ireland, Designing a chat-bot for non-verbal children on the Autism Spectrum, *Studies in Health Technology and Informatics* **252** (2018), 63-68.
[10] K.K. Fitzpatrick, A. Darcy, M. Vierhile, delivering cognitive behavior therapy to young adults with symptoms of depression and anxiety using a fully automated conversational agent (Woebot): A Randomized Controlled Trial *JMIR Mental Health* **4** (2017), e19.
[11] T. Schmidlen, M. Schwartz, K. DiLoreto, H.L. Kirchner, A.C. Sturm, Patient assessment of chatbots for the scalable delivery of genetic counseling, *Journal of Genetic Counselling* **28** (2019), 1166-1177.
[12] V. Fromkin, R. Rodman, N. Hyams, M. Amberber, F. Cox, & R. Thornton, *An introduction to Language.* (9th ed.) Cengage Learning, Australia, 2018.
[13] B. Bosker, Siri is taking a new approach to suicide, *The Huffington Post*, 2017.
[14] https://www.huffingtonpost.com.au/entry/siri-suicide_n_3465946?ri18n=true last accessed 2020-09-11.
[15] B. Carpenter, C. Bond, G. Tait, et al. Who leaves suicide notes? An exploration of victim characteristics and suicide method of completed suicides in Queensland. *Archives of Suicide Research* **20** (2016), 176-190.
[16] V. Callanan, M., Davis, M.A comparison of suicide note writers with suicides who did not leave notes. *Suicide and Life-Threatening Behavior* **39** (2009), 558-568.
[17] J. Pestian, N. Nasrallah, P. Matykiewicz, A. Bennett, A.A Leenaars, Suicide note classification using natural language processing: a content analysis. *Biomedical Informatics Insights* **3** (2010), 19-28.
[18] E.S. Shneidman, N.L. Farberow, *Clues to Suicide*, McGraw-Hill Book Company Inc, New York, 1957.
[19] A.A. Leenars, *Suicide Notes: Predictive Clues and Patterns*, Human Sciences Press, New York, 1988.
[20] D. Ireland, H. Hassanzadeh, S.N. Tran, Sentimental analysis for AIML-based e-health conversational agent, *ICONIP Neural Information Processing* **11302** (2018), 41-51.
[21] G.A. Miller WordNet: A lexical database for English, *Communications of the ACM* **38** (1995), 39-41.
[22] E S. Shneidman, The logical environment of suicide. *Suicide and Life-Threatening Behavior* **11** (1981), 282-285.
[23] E.S. Shneidman, The suicidal logic of Cesare Pavese, *Journal of the American Academy of Psychoanalysis* **10** (1982), 547-563.
[24] M. Fitting, *First-order Logic and Automated Theorem Proving* (2nd ed.). Springer-Verlag, 1996.
[25] Meyer, J.-J. Ch. A different approach to deontic logic: deontic logic viewed as a variant of dynamic logic. *Notre Dame Journal of Formal Logic* **29** (1987), 109-136.
[26] I. Asimov, *I, Robot*, New American Library, New York, 1950.
[27] E.S. Shneidman, Classifications of suicidal phenomena. *Bulletin of Suicidology*, **2** (1968) 1-9.
[28] G. Arsenault-Lapierre, C. Kim, G. Turecki, Psychiatric diagnoses in 3275 suicides: a meta-analysis. *BMC Psychiatry*, **4** (2004) 37-89.

Healthier Lives, Digitally Enabled
M. Merolli et al. (Eds.)
© 2021 The authors and IOS Press.

doi:10.3233/SHTI210007

Patient Flow Simulation Using Historically Informed Synthetic Data

Ezra KENNY [a], Hamed HASSANZADEH [a], Sankalp KHANNA [a],
Justin BOYLE [a] and Sandra LOUISE [a]
[a] Australian e-Health Research Centre, CSIRO

Abstract. Hospital overcrowding is a major problem for healthcare systems around the globe. In order to better estimate future demands and adequate resources for coping with such demands, statistical and computerised modelling can be applied. This can then allow healthcare administrators and decision makers to quantify the impacts of various "what-if" scenarios on hospital performance measures. This paper investigates the application of Discrete Event Simulation towards optimising Emergency Department resources while measuring overall length of stay and queuing time of emergency patients as a target performance measure. In particular, we explore strategies for generating historically informed synthetic data that helps the simulation model track patient flow through the target hospital over a future time frame. Using the developed simulation model, several resource configurations are tested using data from one of the busiest emergency departments in the state of Queensland as the baseline while quantifying the impacts of such changes on key patient flow metrics. It was found that adding a single bed (and associated re-sources) to the emergency department would result in a 23% decrease in average patient treatment delay.

Keywords. patient flow, Discrete Event Simulation, bed optimisation

1. Introduction

Hospitals in many countries are increasingly overburdened, due to the ageing population, increased community expectations, and a higher availability of therapeutic interventions. This causes issues with overcrowding and long patient wait times. Increasing the size of existing hospitals is one solution that can help to enhance patient flow. However, adding extra beds to hospitals in the absence of careful examination of current flow blockages within a hospital may result in additional costs to a health care system without improving accessibility to these facilities [1]. Even after pinpointing the bottlenecks in patient flow, it is hard for administrators to quantify the advantage of increasing the capacity and the impact of such expansion on overall flow metrics.

This paper focuses on applying simulation modelling to analyse the effect of capacity variations on patient flow metrics. More specifically, Discrete Event Simulation (DES) was adopted to model patient flow through a hospital's Emergency Department (ED). Different patient flow metrics, such as patient waiting time and average length of stay (LOS), were calculated to quantify the effects of changes in capacity. A synthetic data generator was also developed that learns the trends in the patient flow of the target hospital using a set of historical observations and can then project such demands over a longer future time frame. This simulation model enables health care administrators to make more informed decisions by having a better understanding of the effect of different "what-if" scenarios through retrospective and foresight analysis.

2. Related Work

There are many examples of simulation applied to operations research in healthcare, to readily and cheaply assess operational scenarios. For example, in a study of an Australian hospital, Khanna et al. assessed the impact of various time-based targets for when patients should be discharged from inpatient wards. They found that discharging 80% of the day's patient output by 11 a.m. resulted in a 16% improvement in National Emergency Access Target compliance [2]. Simulation has also been used to analyse patient pathways and determine the most efficient paths available, as in Kovalchuk et al. [3]. A study by Cildoz et al. used simulation and optimisation principles to find ways of developing priority queues (based on patient urgency), while limiting overcrowding [4]. Olabisi and Nwonye used DES in a hospital context, and, in a similar method to this paper, compared actual outcomes (such as average waiting time, queue length) to those from the simulation to calibrate and validate the designed system [5]. Another DES-based approach by Lal et al. found an optimised clinician schedule by aiming to match treatment capacity to patient load over a typical week [6].

A simulation-based study by Best et al. showed promising results by matching staffing to the patient arrival profile, though this simulation used a relatively small sample size [7]. Ahmed and Alkhamis designed a DES system that allows for stochastically varying constraints focusing on emergency department staffing required to maximise patient throughput and minimise waiting time [8]. As a final example, Steward et al. implemented a simulation to investigate workflow associated with patient care streams [9]. In this scenario, patient journey was determined by their care stream (critical, diagnostic, therapeutic, fast-track, or resuscitation), and the authors found this method reduced both patient LOS and wait time. While there are many DES studies applied to the healthcare field, none report on the use of synthetic data modelled from historical data, which this paper explores. Such synthetic data may allow exploration of system impacts beyond the constraints imposed by observed data. This includes exploring a longer time period or assessing resources such as wards or staffing that are not historically included in the data.

3. Methodology

3.1. Discrete Event Simulation

In large-scale healthcare scenarios, it can be difficult, risky and expensive to experiment with protocols, operational scenarios, and resources. This often means that simulation modelling is among the safest and least costly ways of analysing these situations. One of the widely applied techniques to model systems that include wait times and queueing is DES. Within DES, resources are objects or services that can be used (e.g. hospital wards) with a finite capacity (e.g. number of beds), and the objects of interest (e.g. patients) will

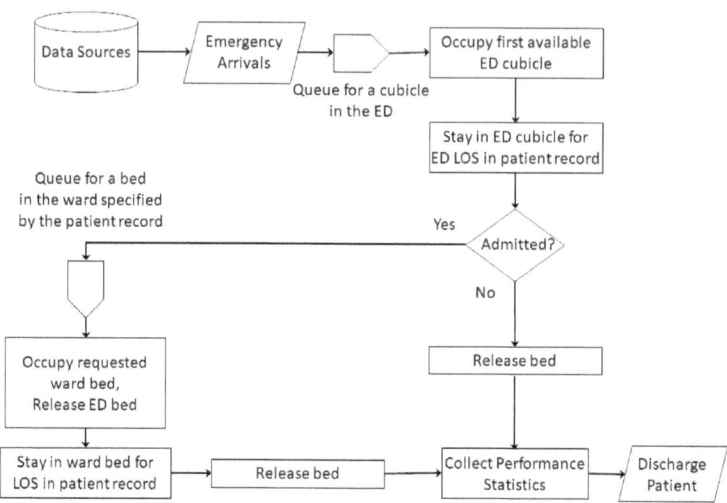

Figure 1. ED patient flow modelling.

queue for desired resources, hold them for a time, and then release them in interactions called "events".

Figure 1 shows the flowchart that was used to create the DES simulation. It involves sorting through the data source to obtain emergency arrivals, which are entered into a queue for an ED bed (this is treatment delay). Once one is available, the patient occupies that bed for the LOS specified in their patient record. Then, if they are admitted to hospital, they queue for the ward they are to be admitted to (this is ED discharge delay). They occupy a bed in that ward for the LOS in their patient record, and then release the bed before performance statistics are collected and the patient is discharged. If the patient is not admitted, after their ED LOS is complete they release the bed, performance statistics are collected and the patient is discharged. This simulation model enables the quantification of the impacts of changing capacities in both ED and inpatient wards (in terms of number of beds/resources), but analysis reported in this paper will focus on the effect a change in ED beds will have on treatment delay.

By giving finite capacities to the resources (i.e. ED beds) in the simulation, queues begin to form once all the beds are occupied. The time that patients wait in the queue to obtain a bed is calculated as their waiting time and materialised as treatment or discharge delays. The priority of patients for receiving treatment services was also modelled in this simulation by considering their urgency level, which was assessed during the triage process.

3.2. Synthetic Data Generation Using Historical Observations

The above-mentioned simulation model can be developed to mimic the historic observations and to quantify the impacts of various changes through a retrospective analysis. In order to enable the model to simulate such impacts in a longer future time frame that exceeds the historic observations, a set of synthetically-generated data should be used. However, the quality of the generated data directly affects the accuracy of the quantified effects returned by the model.

The method of Kernel Density Estimation was used to generate new data. Kernel Density Estimation uses all of the target hospital data, centring a kernel function at each point. Since it keeps the distributions (in arrival times, urgency category, etc.) inherent in the historical information, the synthetic data can accurately reflect the patient flow in the target hospital.

A number of kernels were investigated for this simulation, including Gaussian, top hat, linear and cosine kernels. The Gaussian kernel most closely fit the actual distributions and so it was adopted in our synthetic data generator. The generator was then used to produce patient arrivals on a daily basis. Apart from the admission rates, the generator reproduced several patient characteristics including their Australasian Triage Scale urgency category, discharge destination (whether they were subsequently admitted or discharged home after ED treatment), inpatient admitted wards, and the LOS in each ward. With the actual data as an input, the generator learns the distribution of such characteristics and any given amount of data could be output.

This analysis focused on a Queensland metropolitan hospital with one of the busiest emergency departments in the state, seeing more than 88,000 presentations each year. A de-identified data extract for a period of 18 months (from 1 July 2018 to 31 December 2019) of all ED admissions to the target hospital was used to train the synthetic data generator. Ethics approval was obtained from the Hospital's Human Research Ethics Committee. The data was cleaned to remove any inconsistent patient records, and missing values were replaced with adjacent timestamps where applicable. Patients who died within the ED or who did not stay for treatment contributed to a small fraction of the total patients, and were removed from the data. The details for each patient contained timestamps showing their journey throughout the hospital including time they arrived at ED, were triaged, treated, were ready for discharge, departed from ED and where applicable, subsequent inpatient admission and discharge times.

In order to validate the data generator, a set of synthetic data for 18 months was generated. The output performance measures of the simulation model using actual and synthetic data sets were compared to ensure that the synthetic data reflected actual patterns. Following this, an extended set of synthetic data spanning 30 months was generated, which was then used to report the performance measures of the simulated hospital environment for an additional successive year.

3.3. Experimental Setup

Within the Python programming language, a module called Scikit-learn was used to investigate and adopt a suitable kernel density function [10]. The simulation was developed using SimPy, which is a library in Python specifically designed for DES. The synthetic data was input to the program, which simulated the movement of patients through the ED, and calculated the simulated time taken for triage, waiting for a bed and treatment. The modelling of the priority of patients to receive treatment service was performed using patients' urgency category as the priority value in the SimPy's "Priority Resource".

A number of ED-related performance measures were calculated to quantify the impacts of changing ED bed capacity. These include average ED LOS, and average waiting time before and after treatment (treatment and discharge delay, respectively). The results were also further separated by admitted, non-admitted, and all patient populations.

The simulation model was run with a configuration that meant the ED waiting room has infinite capacity, and the ED capacity reflects the availability of both cubicles/beds and staff. In the absence of a pre-defined ED capacity, the model was calibrated with an ED capacity that resulted in measures closest to the actual outputs.

4. Results and Discussion

Several bed configurations were investigated using the developed simulation model. Table 1 shows results for just one of the ED performance measures assessed: the percentage decrease in treatment delay when increasing the number of ED beds, compared to the baseline (i.e. with the calibrated ED capacity). The results are given for three patient cohorts: admitted, non-admitted, and all patients. The simulated results in Table 1 show two different settings: 1) using 18 months of data, and 2) using 30 months of data. In the former setting, the first 6 months was considered as the warm-up period while the first 18 months was the warm-up period for the latter setting. In both settings, the results were calculated on the final 12 months of the data.

It can be seen that the reduction in average treatment delays were similar for admitted, non-admitted, and all patients as the number of ED beds increased. There was approximately a 23% reduction in treatment delays as a result of adding just one bed. It can be observed that the percentage decrease was correlated to the number of additional beds and a similar pattern in average percentage decrease was exhibited when using the two lengths of data. This reduction can have a significant impact on total ED LOS, especially for non-admitted patients, whose longest waiting time on average was ED treatment delay.

Looking at the two sets of data, it can be observed that the 30 months setting displayed slightly less delay reduction than the 18 month setting, especially on non-admitted patients. This can be due to the increase in the hospitalisation rate in a longer future time frame. The reason that non-admitted patients experienced greater treatment delays during the 30 months of simulation than the admitted patients is due to their lower average urgency priorities, and hence their longer waiting times in the queue for receiving treatment services.

As shown in Table 1, it became apparent that significant changes to waiting times can be achieved by adding a small number of beds. However, it should be noted that adding a single bed is associated with purchasing further medical equipment and employing more staff, which has a considerable associated cost. Although adding 4 beds to the ED may not be feasible, from a management perspective, it is still worthwhile tracking where resources would have the biggest impact on patient flow metrics and when the addition of resources ceases to have a large enough impact on patient throughput.

Table 1. Average percentage decrease in treatment delay with increase in ED beds.

Added ED bed(s)	Percentage decrease (%), 18 months			Percentage decrease (%), 30 months		
	All	Admitted	Non-Admitted	All	Admitted	Non-Admitted
1	23.21	23.10	23.24	22.71	23.21	22.79
2	41.48	41.55	41.46	39.93	41.39	39.89
3	55.54	55.03	55.70	53.72	55.84	53.60
4	66.86	66.17	67.08	64.60	66.96	64.52

5. Conclusion

By analysing data from one of Queensland's busiest hospitals, we were able to find trends and bottlenecks within patients' journeys. A synthetic data generator based on historical observations was developed that can provide de-identified data over a customised future time frame. A simulation was built that models patient movement throughout the ED, allowing for the analysis of "what-if" scenarios. The results of these scenarios showed that with 1 added ED bed, average treatment delay times were decreased by 23%. This rose to 41% when 2 extra beds were added, and further reductions in delay were observed as ED capacity increased.

While this simulation has some limitations, in that it does not individually model staff or waiting room capacities, it produces insightful results for the hospital management team to make more informed decisions. There is also broad scope for further research, including analysis of ED discharge delays, and inpatient journeys throughout the hospital. This analysis could include clustering patients by their pathway, clustering wards with similar functionality to reduce queuing and considering utilisation of resources – 85% occupancy is often suggested as optimal [11]. It could also be useful to find and recommend elimination of inefficient patient pathways, and include specific analysis of elective patients and ambulance arrivals.

References

[1]   Morley C, Unwin M, Peterson GM, Stankovich J, Kinsma L. Emergency department crowding: A systematic review of causes, consequences and solutions. PLoS One. 2018;13(8):e0203316. doi: 10.1371/journal.pone.0203316.

[2]   Khanna S, Sier D, Boyle J, and Zeitz K. Discharge timeliness and its impact on hospital crowding and emergency department flow performance. Emergency Medicine Australasia, 2016;28:164-170. doi: 10.1111/1742-6723.12543.

[3]   Kovalchuk SV, Funkner AA, Metsker OG, Yakovlev AN. Simulation of patient flow in multiple health-care units using process and data mining techniques for model identification. Journal of Biomedical Informatics. 2018;82:128-142. doi: 10.1016/j.jbi.2018.05.004.

[4]   Cildoz M, Mallor F, Ibarra A. Analysing the ED patient flow management problem by using accumulating priority queues and simulation-based optimization. Proceedings of the 2018 Winter Simulation Conference (WSC). Gothenburg, Sweden. p. 2107-2118, doi: 10.1109/WSC.2018.8632323.

[5]   Olabisi U, Nwonye C. Discrete-event Simulation Modeling of Patient Flow in Healthcare systems. International Journal of Advancement in Physical Sciences. 2012;4(1):69-86.

[6]   Lal TM, Roh T, Huschka T. Simulation Based Optimization: Applications in Healthcare. Proceedings of the 2015 Winter Simulation Conference. Huntington Beach California, USA. doi: 10.1109/WSC.2015.7408251.

[7]   Best AM, Dixon CA, Kelton WD, Lindsell CJ, Ward MJ. Using discrete event computer simulation to improve patient flow in a Ghanaian acute care hospital. Am J Emerg Med. 2014;32(8):917-922. doi:10.1016/j.ajem.2014.05.012.

[8]   Ahmed MA, Alkhamis TM. Simulation optimization for an emergency department health-care unit in Kuwait. European Journal of Operational Research. 2009;198(3):936-942. doi:10.1016/j.ejor.2008.10.025.

[9]   Steward D, Glass TF, Ferrand YB. Simulation-Based Design of ED Operations with Care Streams to Optimize Care Delivery and Reduce Length of Stay in the Emergency Department. J Med Syst. 2017;41(162). doi:10.1007/s10916-017-0804-6.

[10] Pedregosa F, Varoquaux G, Gramfort A, Michel V, Thirion B, Grisel O, et al. Scikit-learn: Machine learning in Python. Journal of Machine Learning Research, 2011;12:2825-2830.

[11] Bagust A, Place M, Posnett JW. Dynamics of bed use in accommodating emergency admissions: stochastic simulation model. Br. Med. J. 1999;319(7203):155-158. doi:10.1136/bmj.319.7203.155.

Healthier Lives, Digitally Enabled
M. Merolli et al. (Eds.)
© 2021 The authors and IOS Press.
This article is published online with Open Access by IOS Press and distributed under the terms
of the Creative Commons Attribution Non-Commercial License 4.0 (CC BY-NC 4.0).
doi:10.3233/SHTI210008

Utilising Electronic Health Record Data to Assess the Sepsis Inpatient Care Pathway: A Feasibility Study

Ling LI [a,1], Kasun RATHNAYAKE [a], Tsui Yue ONG [b], Cliff HUGHES [c],
Vincent LAM [c] and Johanna I WESTBROOK [a]

[a] *Centre for Health Systems & Safety Research, Macquarie University, Australia*
[b] *Nepean Hospital, Penrith, New South Wales, Australia*
[c] *Department of Clinical Medicine, Macquarie University, Australia*

Abstract. The World Health Organisation has recently declared sepsis a global medical emergency. Obtaining quality data to establish the evidence on how clinicians recognise, diagnose, and treat sepsis is still a challenge. This feasibility study aimed to utilise routinely collected data from electronic health records (EHR) to assess the sepsis inpatient care pathway. We conducted a retrospective observational cohort study which included all patients admitted to a private teaching hospital between 2015 and 2018. De-identified patient demographic and clinical data were extracted and analysed. A total of 47 sepsis patients were identified based on diagnoses recorded and a review of clinical notes. A surgical procedure was conducted on more than half of these patients (n=25, 53%). Nearly two-thirds were given antibiotics (n=30, 64%), of which 87% (n=26) were administered within 2-hours of sepsis diagnosis. Eighteen patients were admitted to ICU and 13 of them were diagnosed as septic in ICU. We identified some aspects of EHR data that could be improved. Overall, routinely collected data from clinical information systems provides rich information to assess the sepsis patient care pathway.

Keywords. sepsis, patient care pathway, electronic health record, antibiotics, sepsis treatment

1. Introduction

Sepsis is defined as "life-threatening organ dysfunction caused by a dysregulated host response to infection" [1]. Despite medical advances, it remains a major cause of morbidity and mortality worldwide. The most recent global burden of disease study, published in the Lancet, reported that 48.9 million new cases of sepsis were recorded worldwide in 2017 with 11 million sepsis-related deaths, representing 20% of all deaths globally [2]. The first national sepsis epidemiology report shows that motality rate of sepsis patients is 11 times higher than that of non-sepsis patients in Australian hospitals [3]. Addressing the challenge, the World Health Assembly of the World Health Organisation (WHO) passed a resolution in 2017 on better prevention, diagnosis, and

---

[1] Corresponding Author, Associate Professor Ling Li, Centre for Health Systems and Safety Research, Australian Institute of Health Innovation, Macquarie University, NSW 2109, Australia. Email: ling.li@mq.edu.au.

management of sepsis [4]. Obtaining quality data to assess how health systems perform in diagnosing and managing sepsis cases remains challenging.

The ongoing rollout of electronic health records (EHR) across modern healthcare systems presents unprecedented opportunities to harness large volumes of data for analysis to answer important health questions. EHRs contain information such as patient's diagnoses, medications taken, and laboratory test results. EHR data has been used to improve the performance of clinical decision support systems for early detection of sepsis [5]. This feasibility study aimed to utilise datasets extracted from different clinical information systems in an EHR to assess the sepsis inpatient care pathway and identify the potential limitations of EHR data.

2. Method

2.1. Study Design, Setting and Population

We conducted a retrospective observational study undertaken at a 180-bed private teaching hospital in Sydney, Australia. Pathology, radiotherapy and imaging are available on site. All adult patients (age≥18 years) admitted to the hospital from 2015 to 2018 were included. Ethics approval for this study was granted by the Macquarie University Human Research Ethics Committee (Reference No: 5201600379).

2.2. Data Sources and Linkage

Patient demographic data (e.g. age and sex), as well as admission and clinical characteristics (e.g. medications taken, laboratory test results, surgical procedures, diagnoses, and ICU admissions) were extracted from the hospital's clinical and administrative information system. Data sets from different systems were merged using de-identified unique patient identifier and time stamp data where relevant.

2.3. Identifying Patients with Sepsis and Diagnosis Time

Patients with sepsis were identified based on: i) International Statistical Classification of Diseases and Related Health Problems, tenth revision, Australian modification (ICD-10-AM) sepsis-related codes as defined by the Classification of Hospital Acquired Diagnoses approach [6], and ii) the review of selected clinical notes from patient admissions by a medical staff (see Figure 1). The clinical notes were selected if keywords related to sepsis or infection were recorded by clinicians, e.g. sepsis, septic, septic shock, infection, inflammation, febrile, high temperature, blood culture, culture, specimen, bacilli, gram, de-saturating, and pneumonia. This review process identified additional sepsis patients without ICD-10-AM codes recorded. The reviewer also recorded the sepsis diagnosis time if available in the clinical notes. All available clinical information related to these sepsis patient admissions were then merged to map out the patient care pathway during hospital stays. This information included any ICU admissions, ward transfers, surgical procedures performed, antibiotics administered, blood cultures ordered, and clinical measurements.

2.4. Data Management and Analysis

Data quality was assessed across six dimensions [7]. To ensure completeness of the data regarding sepsis patient identification and time of sepsis diagnosis, we conducted text mining and review of clinical notes in addition to diagnoses recorded (as stated in the previous section). The data were likewise checked for the remaining five data quality dimensions: timeliness (represents reality from the required point in time), uniqueness (nothing is recorded more than once based upon how that thing is identified), validity (conforms to the syntax format, type, and range), accuracy (correctly describes the "real world" object or event being described) and consistency (agrees across different data sets, and the extent of agreement between different data sets that are measuring the same thing).

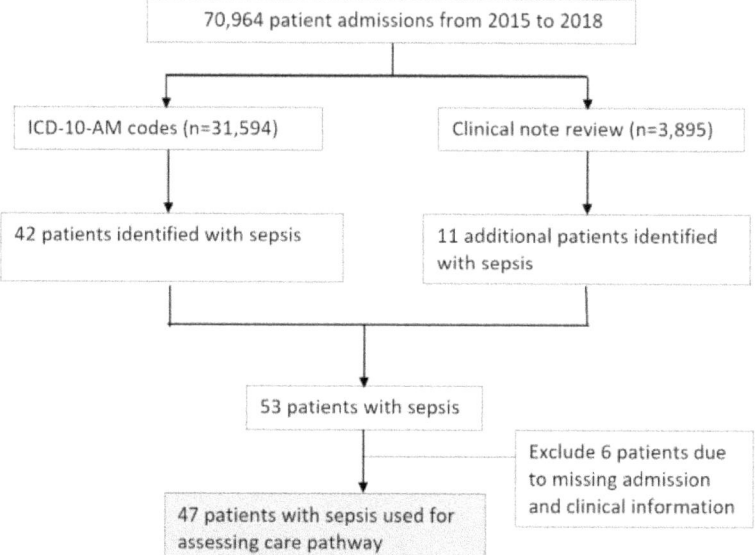

Figure 1. Flow diagram of study population and sepsis cases identification

Descriptive summary statistics were presented to summarise the sepsis patient care pathway data. Sepsis diagnosis dates and times, identified by the reviewer from clinical notes, were used to further examine the sepsis management process in conjunction with other timing information, such as the timing of surgical procedures, ICU admissions, and antibiotic administration. The data management and analysis were conducted using R, version 3.6.1.

3. Results

3.1. Sepsis Patients

There were 70,964 patient admissions during the study period. Patient demographic information (e.g. age and sex), were consistently completed. Clinical information was recorded for patients, including 43,964 admissions with medications administered,

14,356 admissions with laboratory testing results, 21,142 admissions with clinical procedures (e.g. surgery) and 31,594 admissions with ICD-10-AM codes. A total of 53 sepsis patients were identified: 42 through ICD-10-AM coding recorded in patients' diagnoses and 11 based on clinical notes review (Figure 1). Six were excluded from further analysis due to missing admission and clinical information, leaving a final cohort of 47 sepsis patients.

The mean age of these 47 patients was 67 years, and 29 patients were male (62%). Two patients died during hospitalisation. The most common comorbidities recorded were hypertension (n=13, 28%), urinary tract infection (n=11, 23%) and hypotension (n=10, 21%). The median length of stay was 9.5 days (Inter-quartile range- IQR: 2.1-33.4 days).

More than one half of these patients underwent a surgical procedure during their hospital stay (n=25, 53%; Figure 2). Of these surgical patients, time of sepsis diagnosis was identified for 18 patients. The median time from surgical procedure to diagnosis of sepsis was 3.4 hours (IQR: 0.9-21.1 hours).

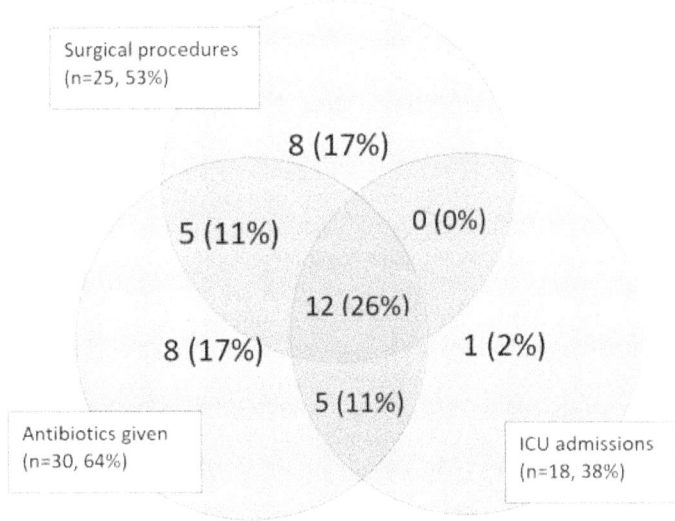

Figure 2. Sepsis patients who had a surgery, antibiotics, an ICU admission, or combination of these factors while in hospital (percentages based on the total sample of 47 sepsis patients)

3.2. Sepsis Patient Care and Management

Eighteen sepsis patients (38%) were admitted to ICU (Figure 2). Among them, 13 of these patients were diagnosed with sepsis during their ICU stay. The median length of ICU stay was 4.8 days (IQR: 2.0-11.2 days). Only one of these 18 patients had no antibiotic administration recorded.

Nearly two-thirds of the 47 patients had antibiotics administered (n=30, 64%). Among them, 28 patients were given antibiotics after sepsis diagnosis: 6 patients within 1-hour of diagnosis and 20 within 1-2 hours. The most common antibiotics used for these patients were: Cephazolin, Vancomycin, Ceftriaxone, Piperacillin, Ciprofloxacin IV, and Dexamethasone. On reviewing sepsis-related laboratory tests, 10 patients had blood culture and other culture tests ordered prior to antibiotic administration, 26 had creatinine tests, 18 had C-reactive protein tests (CRP), and only two had lactate ordered.

4. Discussion

A total of 70,964 patient admissions were included in this feasibility study to identify sepsis patients and describe their care pathways. We retrospectively examined a large volume of routinely collected data from different clinical information systems and found the data sets contained incomplete information in key areas. Firstly, sepsis diagnoses were not recorded for 11 patients, representing 21% of the total 53 sepsis patients identified. These 11 patients were identified through retrospective review of clinical notes. Secondly, this review process identified another critical piece of missing information: the timing of sepsis diagnosis. In addition, six sepsis patients had missing admission and other clinical information Despite these limitations, the EHR data provided extensive information about sepsis patients and their hospital stay, including type and time of surgical procedures, laboratory testing, and antibiotic administration.

Numerous global, national, and local, clinical guidelines have been developed to support sepsis recognition, diagnosis, and early treatment. Internationally, the latest 2017 Surviving Sepsis Guideline panel provided 93 statements on early management and resuscitation of patients with sepsis or septic shock [8]. In Australia, the prominent SEPSIS KILLS program provides sepsis care pathways and guidelines widely used in NSW public hospitals [9]. Our study found that routinely collected EHR data, includes time stamped records of important patient hospital stay information, making it possible to assess patient care, and patient care timelines, against these established clinical guidelines. Antibiotic administration is one of the most commonly recommended sepsis treatments. In our study cohort, antibiotics were administered quickly when given, as per guidelines, with 26 out of 30 patients being given antibiotics within 2 hours of diagnosis. However, the remaining 17 out of 47 sepsis patients were not recorded to have been given antibiotics. Moreover, laboratory tests, including blood culture, are recommended prior to administrating antibiotics. In this study, we found only 10 out of 47 patients had blood culture and other culture tests ordered prior to antibiotic administration.

While much attention has been placed on the identification of sepsis in ICU patients, we found only 10 out of 47 patients were diagnosed while in ICU, consistent with findings from previous studies [10; 11]. Previous studies also highlight the relatively high sepsis mortality rates among the general ward patients, up to 50% [10-12]. Thus, further investigation on the diagnosis and treatment of sepsis in general ward patients is justified. More than half the patients in our study had surgery, which is similarly in line with results from other studies [13].

This feasibility study was conducted at a private teaching hospital, which does not have an emergency department and does not offer a comprehensive range of hospital care services. Therefore, the reported incidence of sepsis might be lower than the average general teaching hospital. Additionally, while the small number of sepsis patients made elements of our study easier to manage, such as conducting chart review (n=3,895 patients), caution should be taken when generalising these results.

Overall, findings from this feasibility study warrant further investigation using a larger population to conduct a comprehensive analysis of the sepsis care pathway after addressing the current limitations of EHR data. Quality EHR data will not only help us to understand the variations in sepsis care against relevant clinical guidelines, but also provide a foundation for designing and implementing an electronic sepsis care pathway to improve sepsis patient care and outcomes.

5. Conclusion

We found that routinely collected data from clinical information systems provided rich information to assess the sepsis patient care pathway. We identified some aspects of EHR data that could be improved to enhance the use of such quality data for comparing sepsis care against current clinical guidelines and for designing and implementing an electronic sepsis care pathway to improve patient outcomes.

References

[1] M. Singer, C.S. Deutschman, C.W. Seymour, M. Shankar-Hari, D. Annane, M. Bauer, R. Bellomo, G.R. Bernard, J.D. Chiche, C.M. Coopersmith, R.S. Hotchkiss, M.M. Levy, J.C. Marshall, G.S. Martin, S.M. Opal, G.D. Rubenfeld, T. van der Poll, J.L. Vincent, and D.C. Angus, The Third International Consensus Definitions for Sepsis and Septic Shock (Sepsis-3), *JAMA* **315** (2016), 801-810.

[2] K.E. Rudd, S.C. Johnson, K.M. Agesa, K.A. Shackelford, D. Tsoi, D.R. Kievlan, D.V. Colombara, K.S. Ikuta, N. Kissoon, S. Finfer, C. Fleischmann-Struzek, F.R. Machado, K.K. Reinhart, K. Rowan, C.W. Seymour, R.S. Watson, T.E. West, F. Marinho, S.I. Hay, R. Lozano, A.D. Lopez, D.C. Angus, C.J.L. Murray, and M. Naghavi, Global, regional, and national sepsis incidence and mortality, 1990–2017: analysis for the Global Burden of Disease Study, *The Lancet* **395** (2020), 200-211.

[3] L. Li, N. Sunderland, K. Rathnayake, and J. Westbrook, *Epidemiology of Sepsis in Australian Public Hospitals: A Mixed Methods, National Longitudinal Study (2013-2018)*, Australian Commission on Safety and Quality in Health Care, 2020.

[4] World Health Organisation, *Service delivery and safety. Improving the prevention, diagnosis and clinical management of sepsis*, retrieved from https://www.who.int/servicedeliverysafety/areas/sepsis/en/.

[5] L. Li, K. Rathnayake, M. Green, M. Fullick, A. Shetty, S. Walter, J. Braithwaite, H. Lander, and J.I. Westbrook, Improving the Performance of Clinical Decision Support for Early Detection of Sepsis: A Retrospective Observational Cohort Study, *Stud Health Technol Inform* **264** (2019), 679-683.

[6] T.J. Jackson, J.L. Michel, R.F. Roberts, C.M. Jorm, and J.G. Wakefield, A classification of hospital-acquired diagnoses for use with routine hospital data, *Medical Journal of Australia* **191** (2009), 544-548.

[7] Data Quality Dimentaions Working Group, *The Six Dimensions of EHDI Data Quality Assessment*, DAMA UK, 2013.

[8] A. Rhodes, L.E. Evans, W. Alhazzani, M.M. Levy, M. Antonelli, R. Ferrer, A. Kumar, J.E. Sevransky, C.L. Sprung, M.E. Nunnally, B. Rochwerg, G.D. Rubenfeld, D.C. Angus, D. Annane, R.J. Beale, G.J. Bellinghan, G.R. Bernard, J.D. Chiche, C. Coopersmith, D.P. De Backer, C.J. French, S. Fujishima, H. Gerlach, J.L. Hidalgo, S.M. Hollenberg, A.E. Jones, D.R. Karnad, R.M. Kleinpell, Y. Koh, T.C. Lisboa, F.R. Machado, J.J. Marini, J.C. Marshall, J.E. Mazuski, L.A. McIntyre, A.S. McLean, S. Mehta, R.P. Moreno, J. Myburgh, P. Navalesi, O. Nishida, T.M. Osborn, A. Perner, C.M. Plunkett, M. Ranieri, C.A. Schorr, M.A. Seckel, C.W. Seymour, I. Shieh, K.A. Shukri, S.Q. Simpson, M. Singer, B.T. Thompson, S.R. Townsend, T. Van der Poll, J.L. Vincent, W.J. Wiersinga, J.L. Zimmerman, and R.P. Dellinger, Surviving Sepsis Campaign: International Guidelines for Management of Sepsis and Septic Shock: 2016, *Intensive Care Med* **43** (2017), 304-377.

[9] Clinical Excellence Commission, *SEPSIS KILLS - Adult Sepsis Pathway*, retrieved from http://www.cec.health.nsw.gov.au/__data/assets/pdf_file/0005/291803/Adult-Sepsis-Pathway-Sept-2016-with-watermark.pdf.

[10] A. Esteban, F. Frutos-Vivar, N.D. Ferguson, O. Penuelas, J.A. Lorente, F. Gordo, T. Honrubia, A. Algora, A. Bustos, G. Garcia, I.R. Diaz-Reganon, and R.R. de Luna, Sepsis incidence and outcome: contrasting the intensive care unit with the hospital ward, *Crit Care Med* **35** (2007), 1284-1289.

[11] J.M. Rohde, A.J. Odden, C. Bonham, L. Kuhn, P.N. Malani, L.M. Chen, S.A. Flanders, and T.J. Iwashyna, The epidemiology of acute organ system dysfunction from severe sepsis outside of the intensive care unit, *J Hosp Med* **8** (2013), 243-247.

[12] L. Li, K. Rathnayake, M. Green, A. Shetty, M. Fullick, S. Walter, C. Middleton-Rennie, M. Meller, J. Braithwaite, H. Lander, and J.I. Westbrook, Comparison of the Quick Sepsis-Related Organ Failure

Assessment (qSOFA) and Adult Sepsis Pathway in Predicting Adverse Outcomes among Adult Patients on General Wards: A Retrospective Observational Cohort Study, *Internal Medicine Journal* **10.1111/imj.14746**.

[13]   [13] A.C.G.P. Elias, T. Matsuo, C.M.C. Grion, L.T.Q. Cardoso, and P.H. Verri, Incidence and risk factors for sepsis in surgical patients: A cohort study, *Journal of Critical Care* **27** (2012), 159-166.

Healthier Lives, Digitally Enabled
M. Merolli et al. (Eds.)
© 2021 The authors and IOS Press.
doi:10.3233/SHTI210009

Improving the Physical Activity of Breast Cancer Survivors Through Fitness Trackers

C LYNCH [a,b,1], S BIRD [a], F BARNETT [b], N LYTHGO [a] and I SELVA-RAJ [a]

[a] Exercise Science, School of Health and Biomedical Sciences,
RMIT University, Bundoora, Victoria 3083, Australia
[b] The Northern Health, Melbourne, Australia

Introduction. Increasing physical activity among posttreatment breast cancer survivors is essential, as greater physical activity reduces the relative risk of cancer-specific mortality. This trial examines how a fitness tracker-based intervention changes the physical activity behaviour of inactive posttreatment breast cancer survivors. **Methods.** Seventeen physically inactive posttreatment breast cancer survivors participated in a randomised cross-over controlled trial. Participants underwent a 12-week intervention of a fitness tracker combined with a behavioural counselling and goal-setting session and 12 weeks of normal activity (control). The primary outcome was the change in physical activity assessed by accelerometry over seven days. **Results.** The intervention achieved a mean increase of 4.5 min/day of moderate-vigorous physical activity, representative of a small-moderate effect (d = 0.34). Changes in time spent as a proportion of the day in light physical activity (-8.3%) and in sedentary behaviour (7.9%), were both significantly different to baseline (t (16) = 3.522, p < 0.01; t (16) = -3.162, p < 0.01). **Conclusion.** Interindividual differences in the change of patterns of physical activity behaviour suggest that only for some, fitness trackers can achieve a change in the level of moderate-vigorous physical activity.

Keywords. physical activity; fitness tracker; accelerometer; cancer survivors

1. Introduction

Physically inactive breast cancer survivors have an increased risk of cancer recurrence, cancer-specific and all-cause mortality. However, numerous observational studies show that being more physically active reduces that risk.[1] Furthermore, increasing physical activity (PA) among cancer survivors is an effective behavioural strategy for attenuating a decline in physical functioning, enhancing the health-related quality of life, and mitigating cancer-related fatigue.[2] Levels of PA among cancer survivors are lower than the population at large. Seventy to eighty percent of cancer survivors are insufficient in PA.[3] Many breast cancer survivors fail to achieve the recommended minimum of 150 min/week of moderate-intensity PA.[4] Therefore, there is a need to increase PA among breast cancer survivors.

The fitness tracker is an emerging and accessible technology that may facilitate behavioural change in PA. Fitness trackers and associated applications have the potential to change PA in cancer survivorship,[5] because they inherently contain behaviour-

---

[1] Corresponding Author, Chris Lynch, *Exercise Science, School of Health and Biomedical Sciences, RMIT University, Bundoora, Victoria 3083, Australia*; E-mail: chris.lynch@nj.org.au.

change techniques, such as goal setting, self-monitoring of behaviour, prompts/cues, and social support.[6] Interventions for PA that have included a fitness tracker have shown an effect in changing PA behaviour; however, for step-count, the effect is only slightly greater to that of non-fitness tracker interventions.[7] Among cancer survivors, interventions using a fitness tracker have shown a positive effect in changing PA behaviour.[8] with trials underway in posttreatment breast cancer survivors.[9] However, with limited evidence, it is unclear to what extent the use of fitness tracker can change the PA behaviour of inactive breast cancer survivors.

The primary aim of this trial is to determine the effect of a 12-week intervention using a fitness tracker, combined with a behavioural counselling and goal-setting session, to change the PA behaviour of inactive posttreatment breast cancer survivors.

2. Methods

2.1. Participants

Seventeen participants were recruited from an oncology outpatient clinic of a major hospital within metropolitan Melbourne, Australia. The trial was approved by the Austin Health Human Research Ethics Committee (LNR/17/Austin/338). Medical oncology staff identified potential participants during outpatient clinics. Participants identified by medical staff or who had expressed interest in the trial were sent an 'invitation' letter. Following a response to the letter, a brief telephone-delivered screening questionnaire was used to check eligibility.

All participants had to be aged ≥18 years, diagnosed with breast cancer (stages I–III), and have completed primary and adjuvant treatments (hormone therapy excepted) within the last five years. Participants were physically inactive (engaging in ≤150 minutes of moderate-intensity PA/week) with no contraindications for PA. Standard screening procedures assessed contraindications for PA.[10] Participants were required to have daily access to a smartphone, mobile device or personal computer. If eligible, the participant was invited to attend an initial trial visit.

2.2. Measures

During the initial trial visit and after giving written informed consent, participants completed a questionnaire recording breast cancer stage at diagnosis and treatments received. Socio-demographic and health characteristics were also recorded. Body mass index (kg/m^2) was estimated from self-reported body mass (kg) and height (cm) using the standard kg/m^2 equation. Participants were instructed how to complete a baseline objective assessment of PA by accelerometry, to be conducted over the subsequent seven days.

Participants were provided with a tri-axial accelerometer (Actigraph GT 3X+; Actigraph, Pensacola, FL) and instructed to wear it on an elasticised belt over the non-dominant hip for seven consecutive days, during all waking hours except during showering and aquatic activities. Written instructions on how to wear the accelerometer and a diary to record wear and non-wear time across the seven-day assessment period were provided. The purpose of the diary was to cross-check data and to refer to if unusual accelerometry patterns were noted. Accelerometry is a feasible method to assess PA in free-living cancer survivors[11] and valid for assessing moderate-intensity PA.[12]

Accelerometer data were collected in one-minute epochs. On return of the accelerometer, these data were downloaded as activity counts. Activity counts represent raw accelerations summed over the one-minute epoch. These data were processed by the ActiLife software package (Version 6.12.1; Actigraph, Pensacola, FL). Data retained for analyses met a wear-time validation criterion of ≥10 hours of wear-time for a minimum of three valid days, with an interruption period of 60 minutes. Each minute of wear-time was classified into PA intensities (counts/min) according to commonly accepted activity count cut-points.[13]

For each valid day, the number of wear-time minutes classified as sedentary, light-, moderate-, and vigorous-intensity PA was taken as the estimate of time spent in these activities. The number of minutes with intensity counts >100 was taken as an estimate of the total time spent active. Counts were summed over wear-minutes to obtain total valid counts for the reporting day. Minutes in each category were divided by wear-time to estimate proportions of the day spent in each behaviour. Daily estimates of the proportion of time spent sedentary and in each classification of PA were averaged across all valid days per participant to estimate the mean proportion of time spent in each behaviour.

2.3. Intervention

The trial was a cross-over trial design. Seven days after the initial trial visit, participants attended a second visit and a Web-based random number generator was used to assign participants initially into either the primary intervention ($n=10$) or normal activity ($n=7$) group. On completion of 12 weeks of primary intervention or normal activity (control) and after a seven-day washout period, participant assignment was reversed. The nature of the intervention meant the blinding of participants, and the blinding of the trial team to participant allocation was not feasible.

At the second trial visit, accelerometer data were downloaded, and a report of baseline PA from the seven-day assessment period was provided to all participants. A motivational interviewing approach guided behavioural feedback and goal setting. All participants were asked to think and record how they could increase their PA and set goals using the report of baseline PA.

Participants undertaking the intervention were provided with and trained in the setup and use of a fitness tracker, a Garmin Vivofit2. The selection of this tracker was based on earlier qualitative work.[14] Participants were shown typical examples of PA data provided by the fitness tracker and application. Participants were requested to wear and use the tracker for 12 weeks and were encouraged to regularly upload and access their PA data via the application. Trial team members were not able to access participant-uploaded data.

2.4. Statistical Analyses

All statistical analyses were conducted using SPSS 26.0 statistical software program (SPSS Inc, Chicago, IL) and performed on the conclusion of the trial. Trial team members conducting statistical analyses were not blinded to participant allocation.

Numerical coding was used for categorical variables. The mean and standard deviation for all continuous variables were calculated. Normality of continuous variables was assessed by Kolmogorov-Smirnov test[15] with a visual inspection of histograms, Q-Q, and box plots. Significance for all statistical analyses was set at $p<0.05$. All analyses were unadjusted.

A paired-samples t-test assessed the effect of the intervention on the primary outcome of PA. Cohen's d calculated effect size statistics and the guideline proposed by Cohen (1988) was used for their interpretation.[16]

3. Results

At baseline, mean moderate-vigorous physical activity (MVPA) was 13.2 (±9.9) min/day, representing 2% (±1.5) of the day spent in this classification of PA. Participants spent the greatest proportion of the day in sedentary behaviour (57.6%, ±9.9) and light-intensity PA (40.4%, ±9.9).

Table 1. Participant characteristics, breast cancer stage at diagnosis, and treatments received.

Variable (n=17)				
Age	(M, SD)	<44 (%, n)	45 to <60 (%, n)	>60 (%, n)
	49.3 (9.4)	35.3 (6)	53.0 (9)	11.7 (2)
BMI kg/m²		<25 (%, n)	25 to <30 (%, n)	>30 (%, n)
	29.3 (6.0)	23.5 (4)	29.4 (5)	47.1 (8)
Months since completion of primary treatment	21.5 (23.5)			
Primary disease stage at the time of diagnosis		Stage I (%, n)	Stage II (%, n)	Stage III (%, n)
		47.1 (8)	29.4 (5)	23.5 (4)
Treatment (%, n)	Surgery/ radiotherapy/ chemotherapy	Surgery/ radiotherapy	Surgery/ chemotherapy	Surgery only
	47.1 (8)	11.8 (2)	35.3 (6)	5.9 (1)
Currently on hormone treatment (%, n)	88.2 (15)			
Experienced menopause prior to diagnosis (%, n)	35.3 (6)			

Post-intervention, MVPA increased to an overall mean of 17.8 (±13.7) min/day, a mean increase of 4.5 min/day. Eighteen minutes represents 2.4% (±1.5) of the day spent in this classification of PA. The increase of min/day of MVPA represents a small-moderate effect (d=0.34). Neither change in min/day nor time spent as a proportion of the day was statistically significant. Change in time spent as a proportion of the day in light-intensity PA (-8.3%) and in sedentary behaviour (7.9%), were both significantly different to baseline (t(16)=3.522, p<0.01; t(16)=-3.162, p<0.01). The decreased time spent as a proportion of the day in light-intensity PA represents a large effect (d=-0.85) and the increase in time spent in sedentary behaviour represents a moderate-large effect (d=0.77). There was no significant difference in vigorous PA.

4. Discussion

The trial was a 12-week intervention that aimed to increase the PA of inactive posttreatment breast cancer survivors, through using a fitness tracker combined with a behavioural counselling and goal-setting session. Post-intervention, MVPA increased by a mean of 4.5 min/day, a small-moderate effect (d=0.34), and a magnitude of effect similar to that of other interventions for PA.[17] While only a small-moderate intervention effect, relatively small increases in PA of breast cancer survivors is associated with a reduced risk of cancer-specific and overall mortality.[18] However, the increase of MVPA is countenanced by a significant reduction in time spent in light-intensity PA and an increase in time spent sedentary. With evidence linking sedentary behaviour to an increased risk of cancer outcomes,[19] any increase of MVPA being accompanied by an increase in sedentary behaviour is a concern.

This trial is one of the first fitness tracker-based interventions delivered to inactive posttreatment breast cancer survivors. While findings are comparable with other trials conducted among cancer survivors, large standard deviations and wide confidence intervals indicate that there are apparent interindividual differences in the patterns of PA behaviour change. Therefore, it appears that only for some, fitness trackers change levels of MVPA but how effective they are, remain inconclusive.

Strengths of the trial include the 100% retention of participants and the assessment of PA by accelerometry. Previous studies have used self-report assessment which may have led to erroneous inferences being drawn on PA behaviour. The use of an objective method of assessment reduces measurement error associated with self-report estimates of PA. Use of an established, normalised equation for accelerometry data, enabled PA to be presented as estimates of the time spent in PA as a proportion of the day. In earlier work, there has been a tendency to fail to examine other classifications of PA, such as light-intensity PA and sedentary behaviour.

The sample size is the substantial limitation of this trial. Referral to the trial was by oncology staff within an oncology outpatient clinic. This approach to recruitment enabled 38 potential participants to be contacted over the recruitment period. However, 20 individuals declined to participate after being further information, and this resulted in essentially a small convenience sample. The sample is, therefore, likely subject to selection bias. The willingness of individuals to participate in a PA intervention may distinguish them from those physically inactive survivors of breast cancer who may not wish to or feel unable to change PA behaviour regardless. Potential participants may have also been dissuaded from the trial by low computer and technical literacy. Additionally, like many PA interventions, the trial was multi-component, compromising of three elements of which the fitness tracker was the primary element. Yet the efficacy of any technique included in the inherent behaviour-change techniques of the fitness tracker and associated application cannot be discerned.

Future work should attempt to identify and delineate the most effective elements of fitness tracker-based PA interventions so that only the most salient intervention components are used with specific participants. Furthermore, future work should be aware of how any increase of PA may be displaced to potentially detrimental sedentary behaviour and include methods counteract it. Use of application programming interfaces, developed and administrated by either the trial team or the fitness tracker manufacturer should also be used to allow monitoring of compliance with the intervention.

The interindividual differences in the change of patterns of physical activity behaviour suggest that only for some, fitness trackers can achieve a change in levels of

MVPA. As any increase in MVPA appears to be accompanied by an increase in sedentary behaviour, future interventions should simultaneously aim to increase PA and reduce sedentary behaviour.

References

[1]   Cormie, P., et al., *The Impact of Exercise on Cancer Mortality, Recurrence, and Treatment-Related Adverse Effects.* Epidemiologic Reviews, 2017. **39**(1): p. 71-92.

[2]   Lahart, I.M., et al., *Physical activity for women with breast cancer after adjuvant therapy.* The Cochrane Database of Systematic Reviews, 2018(1).

[3]   Loprinzi, P.D. and H. Lee, *Rationale for promoting physical activity among cancer survivors: literature review and epidemiologic examination.* Oncology Nursing Forum, 2014. **41**(2): p. 117-125.

[4]   Blanchard, C.M., et al., *A comparison of physical activity of posttreatment breast cancer survivors and noncancer controls.* Behavioral Medicine, 2003. **28**(4): p. 140-149.

[5]   Schulmeister, L., *Technology and the transformation of oncology care.* Seminars in Oncology Nursing, 2016. **32**(2): p. 99-109.

[6]   Mercer, K., et al., *Behavior Change Techniques Present in Wearable Activity Trackers: A Critical Analysis.* JMIR mHealth and uHealth, 2016. **4**(2): p. e40.

[7]   Lynch, C., et al., *Changing the Physical Activity Behavior of Adults With Fitness Trackers: A Systematic Review and Meta-Analysis.* American Journal of Health Promotion, 2019. **34**(4): p. 418-430.

[8]   Uhm, K.E., et al., *Effects of exercise intervention in breast cancer patients: is mobile health (mHealth) with pedometer more effective than conventional program using brochure?* Breast Cancer Research and Treatment, 2017. **161**(3): p. 443-452.

[9]   Gresham, G., et al., *Wearable activity monitors in oncology trials: Current use of an emerging technology.* Contemporary Clinical Trials, 2018. **64**: p. 13-21.

[10] Australia, E.S.S., *Adult pre-exercise screening system (APSS); User Manual.* 2011., Qld, Australia: ESSA.

[11] Skender, S., et al., *Repeat physical activity measurement by accelerometry among colorectal cancer patients--feasibility and minimal number of days of monitoring.* BMC Research Notes, 2015. **8**: p. 222-230.

[12] Tudor-Locke, C., et al., *Utility of pedometers for assessing physical activity - Convergent validity.* Sports Medicine, 2002. **32**(12): p. 795-808.

[13] Troiano, R.P., et al., *Physical activity in the United States measured by accelerometer.* Medicine and Science in Sports and Exercise, 2008. **40**(1): p. 181-188.

[14] Nguyen, N.H., et al., *A qualitative evaluation of breast cancer survivors' acceptance of and preferences for consumer wearable technology activity trackers.* Supportive Care in Cancer, 2017. **25**(11): p. 3375-3384.

[15] Lilliefors, H.W., *On the Kolmogorov-Smirnov test for normality with mean and variance unknown.* Journal of the American Statistical Association, 1967. **62**(318): p. 399-402.

[16] Cohen, J., *Statistical power analysis for the social sciences.* 2nd Edition ed. 1988, Hillsdale: Lawrence Erlbaum.

[17] Bluethmann, S.M., et al., *Taking the next step: a systematic review and meta-analysis of physical activity and behavior change interventions in recent post-treatment breast cancer survivors.* Breast Cancer Research and Treatment, 2015. **149**(2): p. 331-342.

[18] Schmid, D. and M.F. Leitzmann, *Association between physical activity and mortality among breast cancer and colorectal cancer survivors: a systematic review and meta-analysis.* Annals of Oncology, 2014. **25**(7): p. 1293-1311.

[19] Lynch, B.M., *Sedentary behavior and cancer: a systematic review of the literature and proposed biological mechanisms.* Cancer Epidemiology, Biomarkers and Prevention, 2010. **19**(11): p. 2691-2709.

Healthier Lives, Digitally Enabled
M. Merolli et al. (Eds.)
doi:10.3233/SHTI210010

Digital Innovations for Aged Care: Impacts in the COVID-19 Pandemic

Alan TAYLOR, Jennifer TIEMAN and Anthony MAEDER[1]
Flinders University, Adelaide, Australia

Abstract. This paper describes the extent to which remote interaction healthcare interventions supported by digital technology are currently being used, or have recently been newly developed for use, in the care of older people in Australia within the context of the existing Australian aged care system and in conjunction with the COVID-19 pandemic. We place emphasis on those interventions associated with primary care provision, and associated healthcare services such as allied health, rather than outreach from jurisdictional health services and acute care. The primary purpose of this study was to gain an indication of the extent and range of such interventions, and provide a pragmatic commentary on their usage. This has enabled the understanding of some characteristics for success, and drivers for rapid adoption of further digital technology interventions, in the aged care sector.

Keywords. aged care, digital technology, COVID-19 pandemic

1. Introduction

Historically, the role for digital technology in the aged care sector has tended to focus on improving access to healthcare. For instance, the National Health and Hospitals Reform Commission recommended to provide "improved access to e-health, online and telephonic health advice by older people and their carers and home and personal security technology" [1], p. 94. Digital technology has been increasingly promoted as central to the healthcare of older people. The Australian Medical Association argued that "aged care sector needs be supported to adopt modern eHealth systems which enable more effective and efficient patient management" [2], p. 2.

However, despite these arguments the roles in supporting aged care and the extent and impact of digital technology-based interventions remain unclear. This study seeks to establish the extent to which a specific class of remote interaction healthcare interventions supported by digital technology are currently being used, or have recently been newly developed for use, in the care of older people in Australia within the context of the existing Australian aged care system and the COVID-19 pandemic. We place emphasis on those interventions associated with primary care provision, and associated healthcare services such as allied health, rather than outreach from jurisdictional health services and acute care, which are not specifically targeted at supporting the aged care sector.

The primary purpose of this study was to gain an indication of the extent and range of such interventions, and to provide a pragmatic commentary on their scope and usage.

[1] Corresponding Author, Anthony Maeder, Flinders Digital Health Research Centre, Flinders University, 1284 South Road, Tonsley SA 5042, Australia; E-mail: Anthony.maeder@flinders.edu.au.

It was anticipated that this exercise would enable the understanding of some characteristics for success, and drivers for rapid adoption of further digital technology interventions, in the aged care sector.

We first provide an overview of aspects of the aged care environment which influence digital technology solutions and the associated changes in service delivery and care models. Next, we present the method and results for the main part of the study, with findings categorised into 4 themes for digital technology supported interventions, and provide a commentary with some examples for these. Then we discuss measures reported at government and corporate levels which have been undertaken or could be undertaken, to enable rapid and widespread adoption of these types of digital technology interventions. Finally we conclude with a summary of our findings according to the derived categorization framework.

2. Aged Care and Digital Technology

The Commonwealth Government Aged Care Act (2013) sets out a number of objectives for aged care including promotion of the wellbeing and independence of older people (and their carers), equitable access to age care, provision of high-quality care to meet individuals' needs, protection of the health and wellbeing of care recipients, and improvement in the integration of aged care services with healthcare services. The aged care system is large, complex and highly decentralised. According to the Australian Institute of Health and Welfare [3] there were 1.2 million people in 2017–18 participating in the aged care system at a total cost to governments of $18.4 billion. The complexity and decentralised nature of the system arises from the number of service providers and the number of different programs administered: over 5,000 businesses were providing services under seven broad-based programs in 2018-19 [4].

In broad terms the digital technologies used by aged care services fall into two major groups [5]: communications technologies such as the telephone, video conferencing, and many forms of messaging, and technologies used to gather and transmit health information relevant to the maintenance of the health of older people such as remote monitoring. Other distinct groups are technology assisted or supported care using standalone elements such as devices or robotics, and intelligent health information systems such as health portals or online care resources [5]. The paucity of support at national level for widespread innovation and deployment of digital technologies such as these "reflects the wider issue of technology being regarded as an afterthought to service provision, rather than being embedded as a critical enabler of services and their underpinning systems" [6], p. 21.

3. Methodology

This study concentrated on digital technology interventions concerned with remote delivery of health services involving active or passive interaction between a health professional and an aged care consumer, by using some form of telecommunications mechanism and associated control and data management tools. The method used was a rapid review based on public media and literature, primarily grey literature (magazine articles, websites), and a few recently published academic articles. This method was chosen mainly due to the absence of comprehensive academic literature on this topic, as the pandemic has been a very recent event compared with the timescale of research studies and peer review publication appearance. For description and pragmatic commentary on interventions, the chosen target sources were seen as the best option for locating current information on relevant applications of digital technology in aged care.

The search period for the study was 1 Dec 2019 to 15 June 2020, the limited period necessitating use of rapid review methodology. The search strategy consisted of three arms. First a Google search for items that referred to (Aged care AND (Telehealth OR Telecare OR Telemedicine)) was performed, and the Google search returns were scanned for relevant Australian examples. Second, scanning searches were performed over the timeline of interest on ICT and aged care industry online publications and websites (e.g. Australian Ageing Agenda, Community Care Review, HelloCare, Pulse+IT), with chaining of links of interest from those sources. Third, reference snowballing was undertaken on recent relevant government related sources such as submission documents and reports (e.g. Royal Commission into Aged Care Quality and Safety).

Decisions on inclusions were made by one expert reviewer (the first author) and the resulting summary of those was checked by the other two authors. A major limitation of this search strategy was that programs and services which had not publicised themselves or did not describe their program as telehealth, telecare or telemedicine service, were not captured. Given the large volume of exposure that has been given to the use of health technology during the pandemic, and the breadth of discourse around telehealth as a generic enabling technology, this was deemed an acceptable limitation. We did not analyse social media feeds (e.g. Twitter, Linkedin) because a large amount of clutter would need to be eliminated, and because most information of value from those sources is repeated in edited media and would be captured in the second arm. The study results should thus be seen as representative rather than comprehensive, and may have excluded some other types of niche digital technology-based services which have been made available to support older people.

4. Results

Our approach yielded 40 instances of interventions which were accepted by consensus as being within scope. Over half of the interventions were reported as being delivered nationally or in multiple States (23 instances). Of those occurring only in individual States, the majority were associated with higher density east coast States: Qld (5), Vic (5), NSW (4), and SA (3). These interventions were delivered by a total of 35 different providers or businesses: 16 of these were health services providers, 12 were aged care and community care organisations, and 7 were suppliers of technology-based products and services.

Thematic analysis of the search results found four major categories of digital technology supported interventions which were reported as being used in the aged care sector:

- remote consultations for healthcare services;
- remote monitoring of the health state of people;
- support for the independent living of older people;
- communications between older people and their carers.

Four distinct delivery settings were identified:

- self care, people managing their own health care services needs;
- home care, service provider managed health care in people's homes;
- rural care, service provider managed health care in non-urban locations;
- residential care, managed health care in certified facilities.

Thematic analysis results are shown in Table 1 and each category is discussed below.

Table 1. Summary of study findings.

Category	Settings	Technologies	Interventions
Remote Consultations	Self care; Home care; Rural care; Residential care	Video; Telephone; Multiparty videoconferencing	Aged Care and Geriatric assessments/reviews; Specialist consultations; Indigenous patients; Primary care; Rehabilitation; Hospital outreach; Emergency care; Allied Health; Dentistry; Nutrition; Daily checkup
Remote Monitoring	Self care; Home care; Residential care;	Monitoring devices; Monitoring systems; Vital signs surveillance; Mobile phone/apps	Home living assistance; Primary care; COVID-19 screening; COVID-19 monitoring; Smart home system
Independent Living Support	Home care; Residential care	Pendant/alert button; Personal wearables; Mobile phone/apps; Intelligent accessories	Alarm/distress response services; Respiratory services; Daily living activities; Hearing aid configuration
Person-Carer Communications	Self care; Home care; Residential care	Video; Telephone; Tablet/iPad; Mobile phone/apps; Internet voice devices	Home care services delivery; Independent living support services delivery; Care services management; Entertainment and social services; Video captioning

4.1. Remote Consultations

To date the major digital technology-based intervention in aged care has been the application of communications technologies to support health consultations funded by the Medical Benefits Scheme (MBS). Consultations with specialists supported by General Practitioners (GPs) have been the main focus, although in a few cases GPs have been able to undertake primary healthcare activities with residents in residential care. Use of these technologies occurred in less than 1% of consultations prior to the COVID-19 epidemic. At the peak of the epidemic in Australia during April 2020, about 40% of consultations were provided using the recently new items in the MBS enable health professionals to arrange telephone of video consultations direct to people at home [7]. Examination of subsequent MBS data showed that people over 60 years received 240,000 consultations in 2020, compared with 500,000 face to face consultations for all age groups [8]. Only 9,000 consultations to this older age group used video conferencing. Using information from a number of general practices in south-eastern Australia following the introduction of MBS telehealth items, the highest usage rates of telephone or video conferencing were for Mental Health, Alcohol and Other Drug, Dementia or Alzheimer's Disease [8].

4.2. Remote Monitoring

The second major digital technology-based intervention, largely un-funded by government, is remote monitoring of health conditions which enables older people with chronic diseases and other conditions to live independently in their home remain out of hospital. While application of remote monitoring has already been adopted by some age care providers on the basis of evidence for the above benefits [9], it is not yet a mainstream component of aged care. Unlike remote consultations, no government funding initiatives directly related to COVID-19 were provided to address remote monitoring costs. Consequently the majority of the examples identified in this study consisted of wider deployment of existing systems solutions or external third party services, to support healthcare in the homes of older people through the use of medical vital signs monitoring and associated communications. A few new services have appeared which are specifically aimed at COVID-19 vital signs monitoring for those in isolation or at high risk, offered as outreach initiatives by major health services [10,11].

4.3. Independent Living Support

Another area for digital technologies being actively used in the aged care sector for the COVID-19 pandemic to support persons living independently, in home or community settings, and ageing in place under the supervision of informal or formal carers. Options may include access to 24/7 on-call services, coordination of self care and home care, cooperation in management of health conditions, reducing social isolation, and better access for people unable to travel. Many technologies can be employed for these purposes, and sometimes multiple technologies have been packaged into one integrated program. For instance, the 'Staying Healthy Living Well' program is designed to support the health and wellbeing, and chronic disease management of seniors over the age of 70 years of age, via group education sessions using online coaching with a Telehealth Nurse and vital signs monitoring in collaboration with GPs, based around patient care plans [12]. In other cases technologies serve a single purpose, such as provision of alarm services possibly including audio or video interaction. While these types of systems have been in the market for some time, reliance on them during the COVID-19 pandemic has increased due to the higher proportion of older people maintaining self-isolation, or being subject to quarantine controls in aged care settings.

4.4. Person-Carer Communication

While many companies offer digital technology-based human intercommunications and social interaction solutions as consumer services, including embedded functions such as social media or entertainment streaming, there are relatively few products for dedicated care team interaction. One reason for this is the need to achieve interoperability between potentially several different software systems already adopted for independent use by each of the cooperating parties. Another reason is that the business model involves a number of parties cooperating in a shared ecosystem which requires controls over sensitive aspects such as billing, scheduling and information privacy. This requires adoption of underlying standardised information exchange and control protocols, with associated impacts on complexity and expense [13]. Some adaptations of existing platform solutions for COVID-19 situations have been deployed cooperatively by technology companies and aged care organisations e.g. [14,15].

5. Adoption Issues

In this study, two major issues influencing the use of digital technology in the aged care sector were identified: firstly, the need to build workforce capability and user confidence in the use of new practices such as telehealth, and secondly availability and access to physical facilities, information technology and communications resources. A common theme for these issues was a need to develop strategies, policies, standards and regulations to mutually support more effective access to healthcare for older people.

The Royal Australian College of General Practitioners (RACGP) recently identified some telehealth related workforce issues in residential care such as an insufficient number of Residential Aged Care Facility (RACF) staff available, variable training and use of standard clinical communication tools, heavy reliance on agency nursing staff and high staff turnover, staff where English is their second language [16], p. 9. These issues intersect with recommendations for technology oriented workforce reform made by the Aged Care Industry Information Technology Council, including sector-wide national strategy, technology as core in aged care workforce structure, provide opportunities for online learning and videoconferencing and enhance digital literacy, and extend inclusion to informal carers [6], p. 49. Rural practices have responded faster in the use of the new MBS telehealth items, perhaps because they have previously been users of telehealth services [17] which may indicate the importance of confidence and experience in the use of telehealth services. Improving client digital literacy is also a significant need.

The RACGP sees significant lack of appropriate infrastructure in RACFs is a barrier for GPs attending elderly people, including lack of suitable consultation spaces, suitable equipment and lighting, unified medical records [16], p. 6. Other barriers identified are exchange of health information between aged residential facilities and primary care services, connectivity issues within aged care facilities such as bandwidth and signal strength, and access to devices by clients.

6. Conclusion

The findings described above show that technology support for health care and independent living interventions has been deployed successfully across a number of service organisations using products from a number of technology vendors. With the advent of the COVID19 epidemic, this type of remote interactive healthcare support was necessary and signs are that the adaptation and use of technology for remote health consultations and remote health monitoring in particular has increased.

A key conclusion that can be drawn from the findings is that diverse combinations of digital technologies can be developed rapidly and effectively to support the many needs of older people to stay healthy and live independent. Remote consultations, remote monitoring, independent living support, and care communications were all achieved using a variety of solutions. While there are system complexities to be addressed in any new digital technology deployment, the technical aspects are seldom the major barrier to its realisation.

This study also suggests that while significant benefits could arise from increased application of digital technologies in health and aged care, there has been insufficient attention paid to addressing or strengthening the enabling factors. The extent of the achievable benefits will depend very much on building confidence in the use of telehealth technologies through collaborations, developing clinical frameworks, skills and digital literacies, providing appropriate physical, information and communications infrastructure and supportive funding models for services that use digital technologies to assist maintenance of the health and well-being of older people.

References

[1]   National Health and Hospitals Reform Commission, A Healthier Future For All Australians – Final Report, June 2009.
[2]   Australian Medical Association, Inquiry into the quality of care in Residential Aged Care Facilities in Australia — AMA submission, February 2018.
[3]   Australian Institute of Health and Welfare, Aged care, 2019. https://www.aihw.gov.au/reports/australias-welfare/aged-care.
[4]   Australian Institute of Health and Welfare, Services and places in aged care, 2019. https://gen-agedcaredata.gov.au/Topics/Services-and-places-in-aged-care.
[5]   Royal Commission into Aged Care Quality and Safety, Review of innovative models of aged care – Research Paper 3, January 2020.
[6]   K. Barnett, A Technology Roadmap for the Australian Aged Care Sector, 2017. http://aciitc.com.au/wp-content/uploads/2017/06/ACIITC_TechnologyRoadmap_2017.pdf.
[7]   C.L. Snoswell, L.J. Caffery, G. Hobson, M.L. Taylor, H.M. Haydon, E. Thomas, A.C. Smith, Medicare Benefits Schedule (MBS) activity in Australia, April 2020. https://coh.centre.uq.edu.au/telehealth-and-coronavirus-medicare-benefits-schedule-mbs-activity-australia.
[8]   Outcome Health, COVID-19 and Australian General Practice: A preliminary analysis of changes due to telehealth use, 2020. https://polargp.org.au/wp-content/uploads/2020/05/COVID19-Insights-Paper-3-Telehealth.pdf.
[9]   Feros Care, My health clinic at home pilot, 2014. https://www.feroscare.com.au/docs/default-source/default-document-library/mhcah-pilot-full-report-jan15.pdf.
[10] N. Croxon, Bendigo Health first hospital in Australia to use new telehealth platform for COVID-19 patients, *Bendigo Advertiser*, 24 April 2020.
[11] K. McDonald, Royal Melbourne harnesses REDCap for home monitoring during COVID-19, *Pulse + IT*, 4 June 2020.
[12] Healthily, Building the health literacy of older Australians, 2019. https://healthily.com.au/building-the-health-literacy-of-older-australians/.
[13] A. Lyons, Applications for health, *RACGP Good Practice* 7:10, 2017.
[14] S. Cheu, New initiatives keep residents connected during COVID, *Australian Ageing Agenda*, 16 April 2020. https://www.australianageingagenda.com.au/facility-operations/new-initiatives-keep-residents-connected-during-covid/.
[15] Catholic Care, Keeping people together through COVID-19, *Catholic Outlook*, 17 April 2020. https://www.catholicoutlook.org/wise-counsel-keeping-people-together-through-covid-19/.
[16] Royal Australian College of General Practitioners, Submission to the Royal Commission into Aged Care Quality and Safety—Statement of Dr Harry Nespolon, 2019.
[17] Outcome Health, COVID-19 and General Practice, Insights Paper no.2 – A predictive impact model for the healthcare sector, 2020. https://polargp.org.au/wp-content/uploads/2020/05/COVID19-Paper-2-Impact-Model-on-Healthcare.pdf.

Healthier Lives, Digitally Enabled
M. Merolli et al. (Eds.)
© 2021 The authors and IOS Press.

doi:10.3233/SHTI210011

On Computable Expressions of Policies for Digital Health: Use for Privacy Consent

Zoran Milosevic [a,b,1]
ᵃ Deontik, Australia
ᵇ Institute for Integrated and Intelligent Systems, Griffith University, Australia

Abstract. This paper proposes a formal model for expressing policies in digital health. The aim is to support computable expressions of legislative, regulative and organizational policies. The model is grounded in the semantics of deontic logic [1] and in modelling concepts for expressing accountability, specified in the new RM-ODP Enterprise Language standard [2]. An example of privacy consent based on the FHIR consent resource [3] is used to explain the use of these modelling concepts. The example involves multiple stakeholders and illustrates the complexity associated with the use of machine learning and artificial intelligence systems as part of healthcare delivery governed by informed consent policies.

Keywords. policy; privacy; consent; artificial intelligence; ethics; FHIR

1. Introduction

Digital health ecosystem is undergoing significant transformation at present, enabled by new technologies such as mobile devices, cloud platforms, new generation of machine learning (ML), artificial intelligence (AI), clinical decision support (CDS) systems, genomics solutions and so on. The ecosystem is also maturing in terms of the solutions available and new interoperability standards, in particular HL7 Fast Health Interoperability Resources (FHIR) [4] and SNOMED-CT [5]. There are also new proposals related to the clinical and administrative workflows [7][8].

These solutions increasingly require addressing cross-organisational and cross-jurisdictional challenges, the central theme of which is ability to clearly specify healthcare and information policies. This is the topic which is broader to that of information security and needs to accommodate expression of such policies as they constrain behaviour of various stakeholders, individually or as part of their interactions with other stakeholders. Many such challenges arise in the context of future intelligent health visions, while unlocking the innovation potential from health data. In particular, the use of AI in the healthcare context is already raising a series of important societal and ethical questions which we will need to address now, to ensure that intelligent health can deliver on its promise, respect existing norms and more importantly, helping us develop norms for some new issues that are starting to emerge [6].

This paper proposes the use of recently published RM-ODP Enterprise Language Standard (ODP-EL) [2] as a basis for providing computable expressions of policies to facilitate clear statements of constraints on parties' behaviour – including the dynamics of delegation in the delivery of healthcare, from a clinician to clinician, but also capturing responsibility of other parties, e.g. the providers of AI and CDS systems.

---

[1] E-mail: zoran@deontik.com.

Computable expressions of policies are also needed to guide dynamic clinical workflow capability, that would gather and use patient-related information during clinicians' observational and cognitive activities. Such a capability can be regarded as an actor in care delivery, governed by a set of policies and acting like an intelligent agent, sharing collective awareness about ongoing activities – representing the *context* of the care delivery. Context captures many situational factors surrounding the delivery of care for a specific patient, obtained through tests or clinician's observations, and managed using their cognitive models and evidence-based models of care. The context also includes jurisdictional and organisational policies that guide care delivery reflecting patients consent preferences – both from the operational and research aspects of the care.

Next section presents key concepts of the formal policy model based on the ODP EL standard, as a UML meta-model. Section 2 illustrates use of these concepts to model privacy consent policies. Section 3 provides discussion and areas of future work.

2. Generic Policy Meta-Model

2.1. Policy Context

The central part in defining computable healthcare policies is the specification of constraints on the *actions* of the parties who participate in interactions. These constraints are prescribed by legislative, regulative or organizational authorities - defining applicable laws and rules for resources, data or interactions under question, i.e. policy context. For that purpose, the precise semantics of the ODP-EL concept of *community* can be used to describe the organizational or social environment for the participants. A community contract is defined in terms of community roles, their interactions and policy constraints that apply to the roles [9]. A community role can be fulfilled by an enterprise object which can be an IT system, a party (which models a natural person or legal entity), or another community, making it possible to model hierarchical policy contexts.

2.2. Deontic Constraints

There are three fundamental types of policy constraints in any normative system:

An *obligation* is a prescription that a particular behaviour is required. An obligation is fulfilled by the occurrence of the prescribed behaviour. A *permission* is a prescription that a particular behaviour is allowed to occur. A permission is equivalent to there being no obligation for the behaviour not to occur. A *prohibition* is a prescription that a particular behaviour must not occur. A prohibition is equivalent to there being an obligation for the behaviour not to occur.

These definitions have been the subject of standard deontic logic [1], but their application in designing enterprise systems requires explicit association with the agent to which these constraints apply. This is also needed to accommodate an agent's goal-seeking behaviour, which may result in their willingness to violate the policies with the expected benefit of potential future reward from doing so [2]. The way that deontic constraints are associated with the agents (i.e. active enterprise objects in ODP speak) is through *deontic tokens*. These are enterprise objects which encapsulate deontic constraint assertions. The holding of the deontic tokens by active enterprise objects constrains their behaviour. This modelling approach provides a pragmatic means for manipulating deontic tokens, for example, passing them between parties to model delegations, and activation or de-activation of policies that apply to the active enterprise objects in the context of their enterprise interactions. There are three types of deontic tokens: *burden*, representing an obligation, *permit*, representing permission and *embargo*, representing prohibition. In the case of a burden, an active enterprise object holding the burden must attempt to discharge it either directly by performing the specified behaviour or indirectly by engaging some other object to take possession of the burden and perform the specified behaviour. In the case of permit, an active enterprise object holding the permit is able to perform some specified piece of behaviour, while in the case of embargo, the object holding the embargo is inhibited from performing the behaviour (see Figure 1).

In order to support the passing of deontic tokens among objects such as patient giving permit to a researcher to access their health record, the concept of a *speech act* is introduced. This is a special kind of action that is used to modify the set of tokens held by an active enterprise object. The name was chosen by analogy to the linguistic concept of speech act, which refers to something expressed by an individual that not only presents information but performs an action as well. Thus, a speech act changes the state of the world in terms of the association of deontic tokens with active enterprise objects. This modelling feature fits well with the nature of AI-enabled digital health applications, because it can support traceability of obligations of parties (clinicians and AI system creators), according to their broader responsibilities derived from ethical, social or legal norms, as further refined through the accountability concepts, described next.

2.3. Accountability Concepts

Party is as an enterprise object which models a natural person, or any other entity considered to have some of the rights, powers and duties of natural person, for example, a company. ODP-EL introduces two other concepts which are useful to describe many forms of delegation in enterprise systems: *Principal* is a party that has *delegated* something (e.g. authorization or provision of service) to another, and *Agent* is an active enterprise object that has been delegated something (e.g. authorization, responsibility of provision of service) by, and acts for, a party (e.g. in exercising the authorization, carrying out responsibility). *Delegation* is an action that assigns something (e.g. authorization, responsibility of provision of service) to another object, such as the act of referral. It is through this mechanism that deontic tokens can be passed across different active enterprise objects, with one example being a delegation from principal to agent.

There are several other action types to capture important business events in any organizational system, and reflect the dynamics of communication amongst parties, and broadly, active enterprise objects [2]. *Commitment* is as an action resulting in an obligation by one or more participants in the act to comply with a rule or perform a contract. This effectively means that they will be assigned a burden. Examples include commitments by clinicians to deliver safe, reliable and effective healthcare to patients. *Declaration* is defined as an action by which an object makes facts known in its environment and establishes a new state of affairs in its environment. This can, for example, be performed by an AI system (or a party managing it), for example, informing the interested parties about the result of some analysis.

Prescription is an action that establishes a rule. Prescriptions provide a flexible and powerful mechanism for changing the system's business rules at runtime, enabling dynamic adaptation to respond to business changes and new needs. This ability is important in any digital health system, to establish the applicability of new policies reflecting new legislations for example, or after the adoption of new recommendations from AI system components.

Authorization is as an action indicating that a particular behaviour shall not be prevented. Unlike a permission, an authorization is an empowerment. In terms of deontic tokens, the enterprise object that has performed authorization will issue a required permit and will itself undertake a burden describing its obligation to facilitate the behaviour. For example, the authorization for the consumer to challenge AI decisions is giving them permit to do so by the AI system (or its creator/manager) who has the burden to do so.

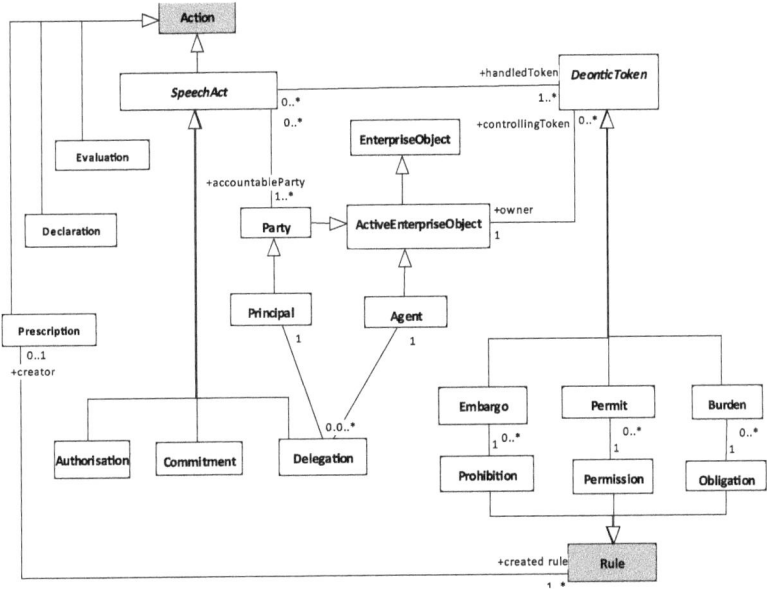

Figure 1. Key deontic and accountability concepts.

3. Privacy Consent Model

3.1. Policy Context

Recall that the policy context can be modelled using a community concept and thus a policy consent community specifies the following community role types (see Figure 2):

- *Grantor,* to be fulfilled by any individual giving consent under a set of permission rules, such as being of legal age.
- *Grantee,* to be fulfilled by professionals with the required credentials, which can be either a *Clinician,* with permission to access Grantors individual health information for care purposes (covered by the patients consent for primary care, e.g. access to all of the patient information in an emergency situation, with certain constraints, such as time period from the emergency event) or a *Researcher,* with permission to access Grantors de-identified health data for research purposes and obligation not to perform re-identification of patient data, as prescribed by National Data Protection Authority.
- *Consent Authority,* a trusted party responsible for storing individuals' consent agreements and overseeing the consent agreement rules; its function can also be to facilitate ethics approvals to govern the secondary use of data.
- *Research Broker,* a commercial entity authorized to search patient health data and consent data to identify patients suitable for research projects. The Broker is responsible to ensure that patient preferences are enforced. It is accountable to the Consent Authority and the National Data Protection Authority.

- *National Data Protection Authority,* responsible for defining and enforcing data protection policies, as legislated.
- *Automated Decision-Maker,* performing analytics, recommendations and in some cases, active decision-making; this role guides and augments activities of clinicians, researchers and other stakeholders, such as population health experts; this role can be fulfilled by clinical decision support systems or AI systems.

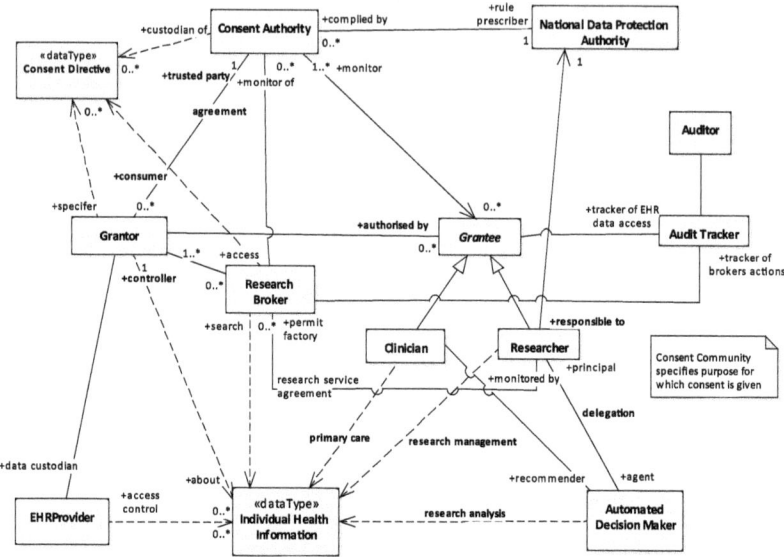

Figure 2. Privacy consent community.

3.2. Deontic Constraints

The privacy consent community defines a number of deontic constraints, such as:

- *Permission* of the Grantor given to the Consent Authority to store consent agreements, e.g. valid for a specified time period defined by the Grantor.
- *Permission* of the Grantor to the Broker to search patients' data and if it satisfies researcher criteria include a link to this data in a data set for the researcher.
- *Obligation* on the Audit Tracker to log data access by the Grantee reliably and on-time and provide access to the audit trail by the Auditor; the tracker may also have an obligation to log actions of Research Broker for forensic purpose.
- *Authorization* of the Grantor to the Grantee to access the Grantor's health information, as per the following actions: a) Grantor issues permit to the Broker for searching their data to establish whether they satisfy research question criteria, b) Research Broker issues a research permit to the Researcher which includes a list of Grantors that provided consent to access their de-identified health data and whose data satisfy the research question, c) EHR provider provides access permit to the Researcher to access health records of specific patients, provided researcher has credentials requested by the EHR provider.

3.3. Accountability Concepts

Authorization is modelled using a combination of permit and burden deontic tokens. For example, authorization of the Grantor to the Broker involves both the permit being passed from the Grantor to the Broker to search its record but also places an obligation on the Grantor itself, through the corresponding burden, to ensure that access to its record is ultimately enabled. This authorization action is also a speech act because it changes the deontic state of both the Grantor and Grantee. The effect of this speech act is that the existing grantor's permit to the Broker to search its healthcare data is passed on to the Grantee. In this example, we assume that the consent directive gives permission to the researcher to access the Grantors health data but prohibits access to the Grantor's mental health data (if it exists). The use of speech acts and deontic tokens is a convenient means for describing the dynamics of deontic constraints and passing of tokens, including to the parties with ultimate legal responsibility. Many data protection rules defined by a National Data Protection Authority set accountability and legal responsibility expectations for actions of researchers involved in using grantor's data. These data protection rules were established through *prescription* actions), performed by the National Data Protection Authority, which essentially establishes obligations and permissions for all the parties involved in accessing patient data.

4. Discussion and Future Work

This paper presents an approach to a computable expression of healthcare policies. This is a difficult problem, but we believe the use of precise modelling framework provided by the ODP-EL standard offers a promising solution path, supported by the use of contemporary software modelling tools. We illustrated this through the example of privacy consent, which demonstrated the expressiveness of the approach, in spite of the limited space available in this paper. In future, we plan to consider applying this foundational policy model to the recently proposed dynamic consent model [10] and consider personalised and fine-grained controls over access to individual information. We also plan to investigate in detail patient's specific consent related to the purpose for which clinicians may use AI systems [11] as part of their care delivery for patients, as well as for providing constraints over analytics applications [13]. Finally, we plan to use this policy model to further investigate ethics and legal challenges associated with responsibility of using AI in digital health as initially proposed in [12].

References

[1]   G.H. von Wright, Deontic Logic, *Mind*, Vol 60, pp. 1-15, 1951.
[2]   *ISO/IEC 15414*. 2015. Information technology: Open distributed processing, Reference model, Enterprise Language, 3rd ed.
[3]   *HL7 FHIR Consent Resource*, Release 4, https://www.hl7.org/fhir/consent.html, (Accessed 7 Aug. 2020).
[4]   *HL7 FHIR* https://www.hl7.org/fhir/index.html (Accessed 7 Aug. 2020).
[5]   *SNOMED-CT* http://www.snomed.org/snomed-ct/why-snomed-ct (Accessed 7 Aug. 2020).
[6]   *Microsoft*, Healthcare, artificial intelligence, data and ethics - A 2030 vision, Dec 2018.
[7]   *Object Management Group (OMG)*, Business Process Management for Healthcare (BPM+ Health), https://www.bpm-plus.org, (Accessed 31 Dec. 2019).
[8]   *HL7 FHIR Workflow Definition*, https://www.hl7.org/fhir/workflow.html (Accessed 7 Aug. 2020).
[9]   Linington, P., Milosevic, Z. Tanaka, A. & Vallecillo, A., Building Enterprise Systems with ODP, An Introduction to Open Distributed Processing. *Chapman Hall/CRC Press*, 2011.
[10] Dynamic consent, https://en.wikipedia.org/wiki/Dynamic_consent.

[11] An invisible hand: Patients aren't being told about the AI systems advising their care https://www.statnews.com/2020/07/15/artificial-intelligence-patient-consent-hospitals/

[12] Milosevic, Z., Ethics in Digital Health: a deontic accountability framework, Proc. *IEEE EDOC'19* Conf., Paris, 2019.

[13] A Berry, Z Milosevic, Real-time analytics for legacy data streams in health: monitoring health data quality, *Proc. IEEE EDOC'13* Conf., Vancouver, Canada, 2013.

Healthier Lives, Digitally Enabled
M. Merolli et al. (Eds.)
© 2021 The authors and IOS Press.
This article is published online with Open Access by IOS Press and distributed under the terms
of the Creative Commons Attribution Non-Commercial License 4.0 (CC BY-NC 4.0).
doi:10.3233/SHTI210012

Automated Inter-Ictal Epileptiform Discharge Detection from Routine EEG

Duong NHU [a,1], Mubeen JANMOHAMED [b,d], Lubna SHAKHATREH [b,d],
Ofer GONEN [b,d], Patrick KWAN [b,d], Amanda GILLIGAN [c],
Chang WEI TAN [a] and Levin KUHLMANN [a]

[a] *Faculty of Information Technology, Monash University, Clayton VIC, Australia*
[b] *Epilepsy Clinic, Alfred Health Hospital, Melbourne VIC, Australia*
[c] *Neurosciences Clinical Institute, Epworth Healthcare Hospital,*
Melbourne VIC, Australia
[d] *Department of Neurology, Central Clinical School. Monash University,*
Melbourne VIC Australia

Abstract. Epilepsy is the most common neurological disorder. The diagnosis commonly requires manual visual electroencephalogram (EEG) analysis which is time-consuming. Deep learning has shown promising performance in detecting interictal epileptiform discharges (IED) and may improve the quality of epilepsy monitoring. However, most of the datasets in the literature are small (n≤100) and collected from single clinical centre, limiting the generalization across different devices and settings. To better automate IED detection, we cross-evaluated a Resnet architecture on 2 sets of routine EEG recordings from patients with idiopathic generalized epilepsy collected at the Alfred Health Hospital and Royal Melbourne Hospital (RMH). We split these EEG recordings into 2s windows with or without IED and evaluated different model variants in terms of how well they classified these windows. The results from our experiment showed that the architecture generalized well across different datasets with an AUC score of 0.894 (95% CI, 0.881-0.907) when trained on Alfred's dataset and tested on RMH's dataset, and 0.857 (95% CI, 0.847-0.867) vice versa. In addition, we compared our best model variant with Persyst and observed that the model was comparable.

Keywords. Resnet, deep learning, automation, epileptiform discharges, epilepsy

1. Introduction

Epilepsy is a neurological disorder in which a patient has an enduring tendency for recurring seizures. In Australia, 3-3.5% of the population is affected by epilepsy at some time during their lives [1]. Electroencephalography (EEG) is an important tool in the diagnosis of epilepsy. Routine EEG records the voltage fluctuations resulting from neuronal post-synaptic potentials within the brain, using surface scalp electrodes. Interictal epileptiform discharges (IED) are abnormal EEG waveforms that are often sharp, standing out from the background rhythm, and are seen in patients with epilepsy. Neurologists use epileptiform transients on EEG to support the diagnosis of epilepsy. Automated IED detection algorithms have received a lot of research interest. A recent

---

[1] Corresponding Author, Duong Nhu, Faculty of Information Technology, Monash University, Clayton VIC, Australia; E-mail: duong.njy1@monash.edu.

review of an extensive number of machine learning methods for automated IED detection (SVM, KNN, etc.) reported sensitivity from 30% to 99% [2]. Among all the existing methods, Persyst [3], the industry-standard IED detection software developed by Persyst Corporation, is the only software with FDA approval and has been shown to have similar performance to skilled neurologists [4]. In recent years, deep learning methods have emerged as powerful computational methods, superior to human experts in various tasks [5,6]. Researchers have demonstrated that the convolutional neural network (CNN) has had promising performance in IED detection [7,8]. However, most of these works only studied a small number of patients ($n \leq 100$). The research with the largest datasets studied 1,051 IED and 8,520 non-IED EEG recordings collected at the Massachusetts General Hospital between 2012 and 2016 [9]. Furthermore, datasets in the literature were collected from single hospitals which might limit the generalizability across different devices and settings.

To address the above limitations, we performed a study of deep learning methods in automated IED detection on a large set of routine EEG recordings of patients with idiopathic generalized epilepsy (IGE), collected from 2 hospitals. As routine EEG is a clinical standard step in epilepsy diagnosis, we implemented a general architecture which was invariant to the diversity of patients. To evaluate the generalizability of the proposed architecture, we trained different model variants on a dataset from one hospital and tested it on the other hospital. We also compared the performance of our architecture with Persyst 14 on a small independent set of routine EEG recordings.

2. Methods

2.1. Objective

The objective of this study was to automate the routine EEG review specifically for generalized IED detection from routine and outpatient EEG recordings whose durations vary from 30 minutes to 1 hour. For proof of concept, we focused on patients with idiopathic generalized epilepsy. As routine EEG is an initial standard step of epilepsy diagnosis procedure, we aimed to develop general models that would be invariant to the demographics of patients, cover a variety of artefacts and waveforms, and would be most suitable for deployment. Cross-evaluation between 2 hospitals will be carried out to confirm the generalizability of the models. In addition, the architecture will be compared with Persyst 14 [3] on an independent set of EEG recordings in IED detection and abnormal and normal EEG classification. We considered an EEG recording to be abnormal if it had at least one unequivocal IED generalized discharge or fragment.

2.2. Datasets and Labelling

We collected routine EEG recordings, between 2008 and 2019, from patients with idiopathic generalized epilepsy (IGE) seen at the Alfred Health Hospital (n = 94) and Royal Melbourne Hospital (RMH; n = 110) hospitals in Melbourne, Australia. These consist of 956 and 1,518 IED, respectively. In addition, normal control recordings were obtained from these sites (n = 98 and 120, respectively). The demographics of patients are summarized in Figure 1. All EEG recordings were recorded with the 10-20 system and annotated by 3 board certified neurologists with accredited training in EEG reporting. We then trained the architecture on one set and tested on the other set.

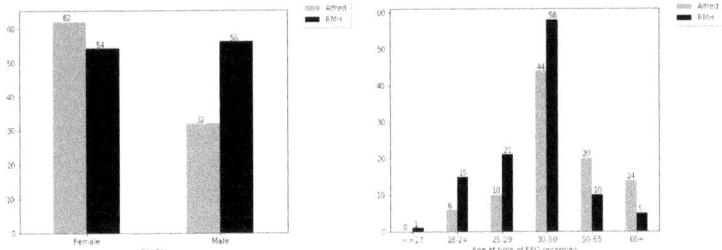

Figure 1. Demographics of patients with IGE.

To compare with Persyst 14, an independent experiment to review clinical utility was conducted with a neurologist at Alfred Health hospital. 8 EEG recordings with generalized IED and 11 normal EEG recordings were randomly selected from 2 hospitals.

2.3. Methodology

2.3.1. Preprocessing

A band-pass Butterworth filter of 0.5 - 50 Hz was used to remove muscle artefacts. We split the EEG into 2s windows of IED and normal with 50% overlap. We used 19 channels and all windows were resampled to 256 Hz. To avoid using any IED, which are missed by the neurologists, as normal windows, only normal windows from normal EEG recordings were used. All windows were z-score normalized.

2.3.2. Architecture Design

Residual network (Resnet) introduces residual connections to overcome the vanishing gradient problem when the deep learning network gets deeper [10]. Resnet has been demonstrated to be effective in image classification [10, 11], and recently in time series classification [12]. In our experiment, we considered each 2s window from an EEG recording as a multivariate time series with 512 timesteps and 19 features, and implemented the Resnet architecture from [12] (Resnet-TSC). Resnet-TSC consists of 3 residual blocks with 3 different number of filters: 64, 128, and 256.

2.3.3. Data Augmentation

As labelling IED is a resource intensive task, data augmentation is a solution to create a variance in the dataset. We implemented the data augmentation method from [7]. In each batch, a reference channel is randomly chosen. The rest of channels are ranked according to the Pearson correlation with the reference channel. This aims to make the model invariant with respect to the location of the channel and keep the local similarities in which IEDs are visible in spatially adjacent channels.

2.3.4. Tackling Imbalanced Dataset

In the collected datasets, the number of windows without IDE is significantly higher than that of windows with IDE. The ratio of IED windows to normal windows from Alfred and RMH are 1:100 and 1:30, respectively. In order to address this, we studied 3 strategies: oversampling, focal loss, and focal loss with oversampling. In terms of oversampling, the windows with IED were oversampled so that the numbers of samples in the two categories were equal. Focal loss [13] was introduced by a research team at Facebook AI Research (FAIR) and shown to be effective in objects detection where background classes significantly outnumbered foreground classes. Focal loss modifies the binary cross-entropy by adding a tuneable parameter γ and a balanced parameter α. The focal loss is defined as $FL(p)=-\alpha(1-p)^\gamma log(p)$. We used the same values as in the original paper for these parameters.

3. Results

3.1. Cross-evaluation Results

We trained the architecture with a batch size of 64. In addition, the cyclical learning rate in [14] was used for faster convergence. The stochastic gradient descent was used with the maximum and minimum learning rate of 0.001 and 0.0001, respectively. The step size was set to 8. Table 1 and Table 2 show the 3-folds results in which sessions were divided into 3 different groups and the results from cross-evaluation on the 2 datasets. The results from our experiment indicated that the architecture generalized well across different datasets. The focal loss strategy had the highest AUC score, 0.894 (95% CI, 0.881-0.907) when it was trained on Alfred's dataset and tested on RMH's dataset. Conversely, the focal loss with oversampling strategy had the highest AUC score, 0.857 (95% CI, 0.847-0.867) when it was trained on RMH's dataset and tested on Alfred's dataset.

To verify if the observed differences among these AUC scores are random, we applied the method of comparison of AUC by Hanley and McNeil [15] with the cut-off of 1.96 ($\alpha = 0.05$). In addition, we applied the Benjamini-Hochberg procedure [16] with the control level of 0.05 to control the false discovery rate. The results indicated that the above 2 AUC scores were the highest and significantly different from that of other model variants within each dataset ($p \leq 0.04$).

Table 1. Results of Resnet-TSC trained on Alfred's dataset.

	Trained on Alfred's dataset	Tested on RMH's dataset
	Mean AUC of 3 folds	AUC
Oversampling	0.936	0.884
Focal loss	0.923	0.894
Focal loss with oversampling	0.940	0.877

Table 2. Results of Resnet-TSC trained on RMH's dataset.

	Trained on RMH's dataset	Tested on Alfred's dataset
	Mean AUC of 3 folds	AUC
Oversampling	0.921	0.815
Focal loss	0.925	0.842
Focal loss with oversampling	0.924	0.857

3.2. Comparing with Persyst

In this experiment, we tested all model variants on the second dataset. We observed that in terms of classifying a whole EEG as normal or abnormal, the Resnet-TSC with oversampling trained on Alfred's dataset resulted in the highest sensitivity and specificity, compared to other variants, 100% and 36%, respectively. The sensitivity was 84.5% in terms of detecting 2s windows overlap with annotated IED.

Sensitivity and specificity of Persyst 14 (at moderate spike detection sensitivity setting) in EEG classification were 100% and 58%, respectively. The sensitivity of Persyst in individual IED detection was 82.7%. Overall, the results are comparable to the industry standard. Results are shown in Table 3. Moreover, we also explored the false positive samples detected by our model and observed that most of them were ocular artefacts.

Table 3. Resnet-TSC vs Persyst.

EEG classification			
Resnet-TSC		Persyst	
Sensitivity	Specificity	Sensitivity	Specificity
100%	36%	100%	58%
IED Detection			
Resnet-TSC		Persyst	
Sensitivity	Precision	Sensitivity	Precision
84.5%	27%	82.7%	37%

4. Discussions

Despite the fact that our 2 datasets are not as large as in [9], we demonstrated the Resnet-TSC with the 3 strategies of tackling imbalanced dataset generalized well across two different hospitals. In the second experiment, we collected a small newly recorded set of routine EEG data and showed that Resnet-TSC with oversampling trained on the Alfred hospital was comparable to Persyst 14. A larger sample size is needed to confirm this. In addition, over-classifying ocular artefacts as IED was found to be a limitation of the model in this experiment. This indicates an additional ocular artefact removal is needed. We will integrate this into our future work.

5. Conclusions

In this paper, we studied a Resnet architecture in automated IED detection on EEG recordings datasets from 2 hospitals. We also evaluated 3 different strategies to tackle the imbalanced dataset problem, oversampling IED samples, focal loss, focal loss with oversampling. Our models generalized well across the 2 datasets. We also compared the models with Persyst, industry-standard software for IED detection, on a separate test dataset. The model with an oversampling strategy trained on Alfred's dataset had the best performance and was comparable to Persyst. We also found that an additional ocular artefacts removal step was needed. Our future work includes improving the models and collecting another dataset from additional hospitals with the aim of providing an interictal epileptiform detector that will be reliable across multiple settings and usable in the early stages of epilepsy diagnosis involving both routine and sleep-deprived EEG.

References

[1]   Epilepsy Action Australia. Help Us Fight the Stigma. Epilepsy Action Australia;. Available   from: https://www.epilepsy.org.au/about-us/for-the-media/.
[2]   Abd El-Samie FE, Alotaiby TN, Khalid MI, Alshebeili SA, Aldosari SA. A Review of EEG and MEG Epileptic Spike Detection Algorithms. IEEE Access. 2018;6:60673–60688.
[3]   Corporate P. Persyst; Available from: https://www.persyst.com/.
[4]   Scheuer M. Spike detection: Inter-reader agreement and a statistical Turing test on a large data set. Clinical Neurophysiology. 2017;128(1):243–250. Available from: https://www.scopus.com/inward/record.uri?partnerID=HzOxMe3bscp=85007206710origin=inward.
[5]   Szegedy C, Vanhoucke V, Ioffe S, Shlens J, Wojna Z. Rethinking the Inception Architecture for Computer Vision. arXiv:151200567 [cs]. 2015 Dec. ArXiv: 1512.00567. Available from: http://arxiv.org/abs/1512.00567.
[6]   Oord Avd, Dieleman S, Zen H, Simonyan K, Vinyals O, Graves A, et al. WaveNet: A Generative Model for Raw Audio. arXiv:160903499 [cs]. 2016 Sep. ArXiv: 1609.03499. Available from: http://arxiv.org/abs/1609.03499.
[7]   Hao Y, Khoo HM, von Ellenrieder N, Zazubovits N, Gotman J. DeepIED: An epileptic discharge detector for EEG-fMRI based on deep learning. NeuroImage: Clinical. 2018;17(June 2017):962–975. Available from: https://doi.org/10.1016/j.nicl.2017.12.005.
[8]   Clarke S. Computer-assisted EEG diagnostic review for idiopathic generalized epilepsy. Epilepsy and Behavior. 2019. Available from: https://www.scopus.com/inward/record.uri?partnerID=HzOxMe3bscp=85074486818origin=inward.
[9]   Jing J, Sun H, Kim JA, Herlopian A, Karakis I, Ng M, et al. Development of Expert-Level Automated Detection of Epileptiform Discharges During Electroencephalogram Interpretation. JAMA Neurology. 2019 Oct. Available from: https://jamanetwork.com/journals/jamaneurology/fullarticle/2752666.
[10] He K, Zhang X, Ren S, Sun J. Deep Residual Learning for Image Recognition. arXiv:151203385 [cs]. 2015 Dec. ArXiv: 1512.03385. Available from: http://arxiv.org/abs/1512.03385.
[11] Szegedy C, Ioffe S, Vanhoucke V, Alemi A. Inception-v4, Inception-ResNet and the Impact of Residual Connections on Learning. arXiv:160207261 [cs]. 2016 Feb. ArXiv: 1602.07261. Available from: http://arxiv.org/abs/1602.07261.
[12] Fawaz HI, Forestier G, Weber J, Idoumghar L, Muller PA. Deep learning for time series classification: a review. Data Mining and Knowledge Discovery. 2019 Jul;33(4):917–963. ArXiv: 1809.04356. Available from: http://arxiv.org/abs/1809.04356.
[13] Lin TY, Goyal P, Girshick R, He K, Dollar P. Focal Loss for Dense Object Detection. arXiv:170802002′ [cs]. 2018 Feb. ArXiv: 1708.02002. Available from: http://arxiv.org/abs/1708.02002.
[14] Smith LN. Cyclical Learning Rates for Training Neural Networks. arXiv:150601186 [cs]. 2017 Apr. ArXiv: 1506.01186. Available from: http://arxiv.org/abs/1506.01186.
[15] Hanley JA, McNeil BJ. A method of comparing the areas under receiver operating characteristic curves derived from the same cases. Radiology. 1983 Sep;148(3):839–843.
[16] Benjamini Y, Hochberg Y. Controlling the False Discovery Rate: A Practical and Powerful Approach to Multiple Testing. Journal of the Royal Statistical Society: Series B (Methodological). 1995;57(1):289–

300. eprint: https://rss.onlinelibrary.wiley.com/doi/pdf/10.1111/j.2517-6161.1995.tb02031.x. Available from: https://rss.onlinelibrary.wiley.com/doi/abs/10.1111/j.2517-6161.1995.tb02031.x.

Healthier Lives, Digitally Enabled
M. Merolli et al. (Eds.)
© 2021 The authors and IOS Press.
This article is published online with Open Access by IOS Press and distributed under the terms
of the Creative Commons Attribution Non-Commercial License 4.0 (CC BY-NC 4.0).
doi:10.3233/SHTI210013

Not Well Enough to Attend Appointments: Telehealth Versus Health Marginalisation

Maria A PINERO DE PLAZA, Alline BELEIGOLI, Alexandra MUDD,
Matthew TIEU, Penelope MCMILLAN, Michael LAWLESS,
Rebecca FEO, Mandy ARCHIBALD and Alison KITSON

Abstract. Temporary telehealth initiatives during COVID-19 have been life-changing for many people in Australia; for the first time Frail, Homebound, and Bedridden Persons (FHBP) equitably received primary healthcare services, like Australians without a disability. However, government changes to telehealth funding mean that since July 2020 telehealth is only available for those who have attended a face-to-face appointment in the last 12 months, thus excluding FHBP. This paper illustrates the reported health exclusion and marginalisation of FHBP. We reviewed the literature and surveyed 164 Australian adults (27% homebound people and 73% affiliated persons) to ascertain their opinions and thoughts on potential strategies to tackle issues associated with FHBP's current circumstances. Results demonstrate that digital technologies and telehealth services are ethical imperatives. Policymakers, clinicians, and health researchers must work with end-users (community-based participation) to create an inclusive healthcare service.

Keywords. telehealth, participatory research, homebound, bedridden, frailty, marginalisation, COVID-19

1. Introduction

Frail, Homebound and Bedridden Persons (FHBP) live with complex, incapacitating, and debilitating illnesses. In addition to functional issues, FHBP can experience financial hardship and social isolation, which puts them at a higher risk of depression (1). Social isolation refers to a state of having minimal contact with other people. It is commonly associated with loneliness, the feeling of missing connections, affection, and proximity in relationships (2). People living with complex chronic conditions, such as older FHBP, require connections, care, and support to maintain their relationships, social activities, psychological health, and activities linked to self-care, mobility, and domestic life (3). This can be facilitated using digital technologies (DT), such as mobile phones, tablets, and computers, which enable remote healthcare delivery (i.e. telehealth) (4).

Ongoing support and guidance with medications and self-care are necessary for FHBP; helping them is a critical public health concern globally (5, 6). An American feasibility study on the use of telehealth for FHBP demonstrated its perceived benefits for homebound people and a reduction in costs associated with their health administration processes and care (5). These findings are important given that many FHBP experience social exclusion, health disparities, and marginalisation from health services because of the Australian healthcare system being devised mostly around physical (i.e., in-person) attendance (7).

As an emergency response to COVID-19, Australia activated a National Health Plan, which rapidly expanded the use of telehealth technologies. This plan included increased practice incentive payments and benefits to allow doctors, nurses, midwives, and allied health professionals (including mental health) to deliver telehealth services to all Australian citizens (4). The response demonstrated that Australia is capable of rapidly overcoming critical barriers to the expansion of telehealth, including well described regulatory, financial, cultural, technological, and workforce impediments (8). As described by Ms Penelope Macmillan, Chair of ME/CFS South Australia (Myalgic Encephalomyelitis/Chronic Fatigue Syndrome) – a disease turning many Australians into FHBP: *"In the past, clinicians only met clients when the person was well enough to attend an appointment. With the introduction of telehealth for GP services, we could meet with them when our symptoms were too severe to allow us to leave home. The understanding of our illness severity and the nature of our impairments was dramatically improved."* (9).

However, on 20 July 2020, without consideration of consumer feedback or needs, access to General Practitioner (GP) telehealth services was terminated for people who had not attended a face-to-face appointment in the last 12 months. The rationale behind the GP-telehealth cut was based on concerns about *"the rise in low-value pop-up telehealth services"* (10). In situations where cuts to services are being considered, decisionmakers must use evidence to determine the risks and benefits of such choices for consumers and consider how these choices might conflict with matters of ethics and values (11).

For socio-technological change and public health policy to be most useful and supportive of the needs of the public, it is necessary to involve consumers in creating and informing such change or policy (8, 11, 12). These participatory research (PR) strategies are required in the system-level change and knowledge creation process (e.g., co-design), in which consumers are included in offering their perspectives and interpretations concerning studies and resulting policies (7, 8, 11, 12). Therefore, with an emphasis on a PR approach, this paper aims to explore the key strategies to tackle the pressing issues associated with FHBPs' described circumstances. The study has two objectives: 1) Provide evidence to inform decision making, health practice, and health research in this field, and 2) Explore consumer-centric solutions that address the problems of social isolation, marginalisation, and needs of FHBP.

2. Method

This paper reports on the first part of a program of research concerning FHBP in Australia: *'Making the invisible visible: Exploring the experiences of frail, homebound and bedridden people'*. The study is approved by the Flinders University Social and Behavioural Research Ethics Committee (Project No. 8557). This paper presents a mixed-method, consumer-centric approach (co-designed with one health consumer as a co-researcher at a peer level with the academic investigators and her FHBP peer-reference networks). The method involves two steps:

First step: A rapid scoping review with the aims of identifying existing interventions enhanced by technologies that target social isolation reduction for older adults. The search is focused on previous reviews (Pubmed/Medline), and grey literature (Google/Google Scholar). The results were presented narratively and classified according to the main risk factor addressed by each intervention as per the Framework for Isolation for adults over 50 of the AARP Foundation (34), published between April 2014 and April 2020.

Second step: Two questions from a larger online survey (Project No. 8557) were selected to explore the needs of FHBP and solutions/actions to the pressing issues they routinely experience (e.g. social isolation and telehealth; the GP-telehealth cut occurred near the end of data collection). The survey was shared via social media as a press release across different universities platforms and consumers advocate groups.

The first question of the survey: *"Excluding an accident or temporary illness, are you permanently unable to leave your home?"* distinguished homebound people (using the American Medicare classification for homebound persons as those whose absences from home are infrequent, or for periods of relatively short duration, or to receive medical treatment, 13) from their affiliates (e.g. people experiencing similar conditions, people caring for FHBP or people invested in the issues of FHBP). The second question: *"Please, check the boxes that you consider important to help you or other Australians who are facing similar problems to yours"* involved multiple selection options about issues with healthcare access. This question facilitated problem identification without demanding much writing from respondents. The list of co-designed options (presented in the survey as potential needs or required solutions or actions) is presented in Table 2. Data were collected from 02/07/2020 until 05/07/2020. Basic descriptive statistics and crosstabulation of variables were used to analyse the data.

3. Results

Rapid review: our search retrieved five reviews. The content of reviews is synthesised in Table 1, which outlines risk factors for social isolation, the strategy and technology utilised to overcome these risks, and the examples or comments concerning each publication (as per 34). The evidence in Table 1 demonstrates that current practices and knowledge can be effectively operationalised using digital and similar technologies (e.g. wearables, systems mapping, social media and robots) to mitigate and prevent loneliness and social isolation in older adults with complex health issues. Such knowledge can arguably be adapted to support FHBP living in Australia.

Table 1. Examples of technologies used to mitigate and prevent loneliness and social isolation in older adults.

Risk factor	Strategy	Technology	Examples/Comments
Living alone	Informational social support (Education/empowerment)	Telehealth (14, 15)	Videoconference groups mediated by health providers focusing on education about health issues led to an improvement in social isolation.
	Increasing social network	Telehealth (16)	Videoconference delivered by lay providers during meals.
	An increasing sense of presence/companionship	Embodied conversational agent (17)	Virtual pet therapy
	The increasing frequency of social contacts	An online platform (18)	A platform that matches people who want to donate meals to ones who are

Risk factor	Strategy	Technology	Examples/Comments
			searching for companionship during meals
	Detecting loneliness and activating family support	Wearable/telemonitoring (19)	Monitoring of conversations and word count throughout the day then prompting social contact when levels drop too low.
Small social network and/or inadequate social support	Promoting integration within local communities	Online platforms/websites (20, 21, 22)	Information-based intervention that provides personalised information and referral service to increase older adults' awareness and knowledge of the services and activities available to them.
			Advice on community events. Focused on older adults.
			Focused on culturally and linguistically diverse people
	Promoting integration within local communities	Geographic information system mapping (23)	Simple map to find community organisations. Focused on older adults
	Promoting integration within local communities	Telephone-based (24)	A resource that provides older men with opportunities for mateship, and the chance to re-connect with the community
	Facilitating integration within families	Home telehealth and telemonitoring combined with social media (25)	Home telehealth system from the provision of health care to enhancing older adults' interpersonal communication and social participation
	Peer support	Online social network/social media (26)	Social media moderated by health professionals
	Promoting structured social support (social network with volunteers rather than acquaintances/friends)	Telehealth (27)	Health provider train volunteers for conversation facilitation. Once trained volunteers facilitate group discussion utilising teleconferencing.
	Increase opportunities for social contact	Digital games (28)	Opportunities for meeting friends online through games communities for older adults
Major life transitions	Emotional support	Telehealth/telephone-based (29)	Online/telephone advice on how to cope positively with life after loss.
Mobility or sensory impairment	Increase sense of presence/companionship	Embodied conversational agents/avatars (30)	Full-bodied gesture-based interactions and avatars can be used to create a sense of virtual presence between older people who are unable to meet face-to-face.
	Increase sense of social participation	Virtual and augmented reality (31)	Overcoming social isolation through the power

Risk factor	Strategy	Technology	Examples/Comments
			of virtual reality and shared experiences. Focused on older adults.
Mental health condition	Peer support	Online chat forum/social media (32)	Focused on people with alcohol and drugs addiction
Cognitive impairment	Facilitate communication with carers	Telepresence robots (33)	Focused on people with dementia

Survey: According to the responses from 164 Australians adults, 27% of whom are homebound and 73% representing their affiliates, the five most important needs/actions to help them or other Australians who are facing similar problems are:

- Education for all health professionals and service providers about people with their needs (96%)
- Educating Centrelink, NDIS, and government services about paperwork difficulties (e.g. providing more time or accepting GP reports rather than specialist paperwork only) (93%)
- Access to community care services (e.g. NDIS, Aged Care packages) (93%)
- Adequate Medicare rebates for home visits (93%)
- Extending the existing telephone or online consults (Telehealth) for rural and remote patients to also cover patients who are housebound or bedbound (93%).

The responses from FHBP affiliates were consistent with the importance rankings of homebound respondents. The relevancy of the needs/action list was validated, with most options checked by homebound adults and their affiliates in high percentages (above 64%).

Table 2. Important actions to help FHBP according to homebound/affiliates.

Important actions (needs) to help you or other Australians who are facing similar problems to yours	Homebound	Affiliates	Total
Education for all health professionals and service providers about people with your needs	43	89	132
Educating Centrelink, NDIS, and government services about paperwork difficulties, e.g. providing more time or accepting GP reports rather than specialist paperwork only	42	86	128
Access to community care services, for example, NDIS, Aged Care packages	42	82	124
Adequate Medicare rebates for home visits	42	81	123
Extending the existing telephone or online consults (Telehealth) for rural and remote patients to also cover patients who are housebound or bedbound	42	79	121
Telephone consults	40	72	112
Ability to fund the testing and medical reports required to access benefits	39	80	119
Regular home access to a general practitioner	39	71	110
Access to advocacy services (including legal) to assist with the day to day issues (e.g. NDIS access, DSP access, discrimination, access to insurance policies, domestic violence, etc.)	37	80	117
Home access to psychology (or psychological) services	37	72	109
Find out about how many Australians are living with similar problems to yours to generate faster solutions	37	67	104
Services to enable you to keep living in the community	35	75	110
Access to housing or accommodation arrangements	35	53	88
Access to food services (e.g. Meals on Wheels)	33	66	99

Important actions (needs) to help you or other Australians who are facing similar problems to yours	Homebound	Affiliates	Total
Access to services that are equivalent to the help provided by home palliative care services, for example, regular home visits by a nurse or GP	32	63	95
Streamlining easier access to patient transport	29	53	82
Other	12	27	39
Total Count	45	119	164

4. Discussion and Conclusion

Our rapid review found sufficient evidence to support the use of effective technological, social and health interventions to mitigate some of the negative experiences of FHBP (i.e. concerning health, technology, social isolation, and loneliness). Technology enables strategies to increase informational/educational support, connection/network or social contact, family contact, emotional assistance, and patient-carers communication. These findings are backed and complemented by our survey findings, in which is evident that technology must be combined with a person-centred approach and a culture of care service that gives visibility to the needs and voices of marginalised FHBP in Australia.

Our survey indicates that prompt action is required to educate all health professionals and service providers about FHBP; educate Centrelink, NDIS, and government services about the difficulties FHBP are facing; facilitate access to community care services (e.g., NDIS, aged care packages); provide adequate Medicare rebates for home visits, and extend the existing telephone or online consults (Telehealth) for rural and remote patients to also cover FHBP in city locations (as it was done for everyone temporarily because of the first wave of COVID-19).

The academic literature, the communities we surveyed, and public opinion (e.g. news media reports), all points to the same direction: telehealth and digital technologies are effective and needed tools to combat the health marginalisation of Australia's FHBP. The task now is to educate several service providers and policymakers about the devastating consequences of maintaining a healthcare system working around the exclusory and impractical requirement of physical attendance. The negative health and psychosocial impacts of COVID-19 are highlighting the relevancy of our findings particularly concerning the groups comprising a greater proportion of FHBP, such as older people with co-morbidities and individuals living with disabilities.

References

[1]   Choi, N. G., Teeters, M., Perez, L., Farar, B. and Thompson, D. (2010). Severity and correlates of depressive symptoms among recipients of Meals on Wheels: Age, gender, racial/ethnic difference. Aging & Mental Health 14(2): 145–154.

[2]   J. De Jong Gierveld, T.G. Van Tilburg, P.A. Dykstra. Loneliness and social isolation. D. Perlman, A. Vangelisti (Eds.), The Cambridge Handbook of Personal Relationships, Cambridge University Press, Cambridge (2006), pp. 485-500.

[3]   Abdi, S., Spann, A., Borilovic, J., de Witte, L., & Hawley, M. (2019). Understanding the care and support needs of older people: a scoping review and categorisation using the WHO international classification of functioning, disability and health framework (ICF). BMC geriatrics, 19(1), 195.

[4]   Commonwealth of Australia | Department of Health. (2020). COVID-19 National Health Plan – Primary Care Package – MBS Telehealth Services and Increased Practice Incentive Payments. Accessed 16.04.2020.

[5]   Choi, Namkee G, Hegel, Mark T, Marti, C Nathan, Marinucci, Mary Lynn, Sirrianni, Leslie, & Bruce, Martha L. (2014). Telehealth Problem-Solving Therapy for Depressed Low-Income Homebound Older Adults. American Journal of Geriatric Psychiatry., 22(3), 263-271.

[6]   Lee, JuHee and Suh, Yujin and Kim, Yielin, Multidimensional Factors Affecting Homebound Older Adults: A Systematic Review (2020). Preprint with The Lancet. Accessed 16.04.2020.

[7]   Buchanan, R. (2018). "Just Invisible" Medical Access Issues For Homebound/Bedridden Persons. Accessed on the 20/06/2019.

[8]   Jang-Jaccard, J., Nepal, S., Alem, L., & Li, J. (2014). Barriers for delivering telehealth in rural Australia: a review based on Australian trials and studies. Telemedicine and e-Health, 20(5), 496-504.

[9]   Disability Insider. Telehealth cuts see services withdrawn to Australians with disabilities (2020). Coronavirus Pandemic, Disability Insider. Accessed 29/07/2020.

[10]   Tsirtsakis, A. Government restricts telehealth MBS access to a patient's regular GP. NewsGP -The Royal Australian College of General Practitioners. Accessed 10/07/2020.

[11]   Solomon, M. Z., Gusmano, M. K., & Maschke, K. J. (2016). The ethical imperative and moral challenges of engaging patients and the public with evidence. Health Affairs, 35(4), 583-589.

[12]   Slattery, P., Saeri, A. K., & Bragge, P. (2020). Research co-design in health: a rapid overview of reviews. Health Research Policy and Systems, 18(1), 17.

[13]   Talaga, S. R. (2013). Medicare home health benefit primer: Benefit basics and issues. Library of Congress, Congressional Research Service. March (accessed on the 20 of July 2019).

[14]   Banbury A, Chamberlain D, Nancarrow S, Dart J, Gray L, Parkinson L. Can videoconferencing affect older people's engagement and perception of their social support in long-term conditions management: a social network analysis from the Telehealth Literacy Project. Health Soc Care Community. 2017;25(3):938-950. doi:10.1111/hsc.12382.

[15]   Banbury A, Nancarrow S, Dart J, et al. Adding value to remote monitoring: Co-design of a health literacy intervention for older people with chronic disease delivered by telehealth - The telehealth literacy project. Patient Educ Couns. 2020;103(3):597-606. doi:10.1016/j.pec.2019.10.005.

[16]   Banbury A, Nancarrow S, Dart J, et al. Adding value to remote monitoring: Co-design of a health literacy intervention for older people with chronic disease delivered by telehealth - The telehealth literacy project. Patient Educ Couns. 2020;103(3):597-606. doi:10.1016/j.pec.2019.10.005.

[17]   Machesney D, Wexler SS, Chen T, Coppola JF. Gerontechnology Companion: Virtual pets for dementia patients: IEEE; 2014 Presented at Systems, Applications and Technology Conference (LISAT), 2014 IEEE Long Island; 2-2 May 2014; New York p. 1-3.

[18]   Casserole Club. Available at https://www.casseroleclub.com/. Accessed on 13th July, 2020.

[19]   Wearable tech lends an ear to lonely elderly. Available at: https://www.rmit.edu.au/news/all-news/2019/feb/wearable-tech-lonely-elderly. Accessed on 13th July, 2020.

[20]   Seniors Enquiry Line. Available at: https://seniorsenquiryline.com.au/. Accessed on 13th July, 2020.

[21]   Connect to new possibilities without leaving home. Available at: https://www.mather.com/neighborhood-programs/telephone-topics Accessed on 13th July, 2020.

[22]   Mosaic Seniors. Available at: https://www.mosaicbc.org/services/settlement/seniors/ Accessed on 13th July, 2020.

[23]   Be Connected Partner Map. Available at: https://beconnected.esafety.gov.au/find-local-help Accessed on 13th July, 2020.

[24]   TomNet – The older men network. Available at: Tomnet.org.au Accessed on 13th July, 2020.

[25]   Yu-Chen Huang, Yeh-Liang Hsu, Social networking-based personal home telehealth system: A pilot study, Journal of Clinical Gerontology and Geriatrics, Volume 5, Issue 4, 2014, Pages 132-139, ISSN 2210-8335, https://doi.org/10.1016/j.jcgg.2014.05.004.

[26]   Beyond Blue. Online social community. Available at https://www.beyondblue.org.au/get-support/online-forums/community-rules. Accessed on 13th July, 2020.

[27]   Brotherhood of St Laurence. Available at: https://www.bsl.org.au/ Accessed on 13th July, 2020.

[28]   Australian Government. Be Connected. Games centre for mouse and keyboard. Available at https://beconnected.esafety.gov.au/games/games-centre Accessed on 13th July, 2020.

[29]   TomNet – The older men network. Available at: Tomnet.org.au Accessed on 13th July, 2020.

[30]   The University of Melbourne. Ageing and Avatars. Available at: https://socialnui.unimelb.edu.au/research/ageing-avatars/ Accessed on 13th July, 2020.

[31]   Rendever. Available at: https://rendever.com/ Accessed on 13th July, 2020.

[32]   Alcohol and Drugs. Counselling online forums. Available at: https://forum.counsellingonline.org.au/index.php Accessed on 13th July, 2020.

[33]   Moyle W, Arnautovska U, Ownsworth T, Jones C. Potential of telepresence robots to enhance social connectedness in older adults with dementia: an integrative review of feasibility. Int Psychogeriatr. 2017;29(12):1951-1964. doi:10.1017/S1041610217001776.

[34] AARP Foundation Frameworks for Isolation in adults over 50. Available at https://www.aarp.org/content/dam/aarp/aarp_foundation/2012_PDFs/AARP-Foundation-Isolation-Framework-Report.pdf [Acessed on 17th April, 2020].

Healthier Lives, Digitally Enabled
M. Merolli et al. (Eds.)
© 2021 The authors and IOS Press.
This article is published online with Open Access by IOS Press and distributed under the terms
of the Creative Commons Attribution Non-Commercial License 4.0 (CC BY-NC 4.0).
doi:10.3233/SHTI210014

Improving the Digital Capabilities of Australia's Health Workforce: The National Digital Health Workforce and Education Roadmap

Leanna WOODS [a], Shiva SHARIF BIDABADI [a], Angela RYAN [a,1],
Tim SHAW [b,c] and Meredith MAKEHAM [a,c]
[a] *Australian Digital Health Agency, Sydney, NSW, Australia*
[b] *Digital Health Cooperative Research Centre, Sydney, NSW, Australia*
[c] *University of Sydney, Sydney, NSW, Australia*

Abstract. There is a need to improve the digital capabilities of the health workforce through training and education. Until now there has not been a national strategy that addresses the digital capability gaps in the existing and emerging health workforce. This paper describes the development of a national strategy to improve the digital capabilities of Australia's health workforce. A mixed-method approach was used to incorporate the findings of a literature review, stakeholder interviews, online and offline workshops, consumer interviews, and surveys to develop the national strategy. Various stakeholder groups across all Australian jurisdictions were engaged in its development. The final strategy consists of key principles, a three-horizon framework reflecting the maturity levels, and a digital profile framework articulating the expectations of the many stakeholders in health.

Keywords. digital health, strategy, workforce development, education

1. Introduction

The benefits of digital health technologies are significant and compelling. Used effectively, digital health technologies can save lives, as well as improve the health and wellbeing of all Australians [1]. Further, these technologies can support a sustainable health system that delivers safe, high quality, and effective health services [2].

Health leaders of today are faced with opportunities and challenges from an array of emerging technologies. These technologies are already profoundly changing the way healthcare is delivered, impacting traditional approaches to health occupations, tasks and functions. A confident and capable health workforce is required to realise the benefits of digital health technologies [1]. Significant investments to modernise health service delivery are being made. All Australian states and territories, and many healthcare providers, have prioritised digital health to improve service delivery and health outcomes.

This paper describes Australia's National Digital Health Workforce and Education Roadmap (the roadmap), which provides a framework for understanding the digital

---

[1] Corresponding Author, Angela Ryan, Australian Digital Health Agency, Level 25, 175 Liverpool St, @000, NSW, Australia; E-mail: workforce@digitalhealth.gov.au.

capability requirements for the health workforce. The roadmap anticipates how the application of digital technologies in health is likely to impact the workforce and education requirements in the short to medium term. It sets out a vision for how the workforce can be transformed over the next decade and beyond to realise the benefits promised by digital health technologies.

2. Background

Globally, much of the focus on digital health remains on the role of existing and emerging technologies, rather than the capabilities required for the workforce to use them effectively. This is despite the significant health workforce impacts that are already being experienced, and those that are being anticipated.

The United Kingdom has released the greatest number of health workforce publications in this area, most notably the Topol Report in 2019 [3]. Many countries are facing common challenges in the implementation of digital health services. In recent years, collaborations such as the Global Digital Health Partnership [4] have emerged in an effort to support governments and health system reformers to improve the health and wellbeing of their citizens through the best use of evidence-based digital technologies. Despite leadership and collaboration in digital health, very few health-specific digital capability and digital literacy frameworks have been developed internationally.

In Australia, while there are some innovative examples [5, 6], the digital health capability of the workforce is still emerging as an area of focus in the health, education and training sectors. The pressing need for recognised digital health training and education is supported by Australia's National Digital Health Strategy [1]. The Australian Digital Health Agency is tasked with implementing the strategy, in collaboration with the broader health sector, including the 'Workforce and Education' priority to support a 'workforce confidently using digital health technologies to deliver health and care' [1].

3. Methods

The roadmap was developed with wide stakeholder engagement and collaboration across the health and education sector in Australia, including a governance group to ensure appropriate oversight. Key activities included the following:

- Literature review
- Stakeholder interviews
- Consumer interviews
- Workshops
- Surveys

Public consultation culminated in the National Workforce and Education Summit, which was hosted by the Australian Digital Health Agency and the Digital Health Cooperative Research Centre in November 2019. Summit participants included representatives from federal, state and territory governments, consumer and clinical peaks, university and vocational education providers, researchers, primary health networks, clinicians, consumers and industry. Many summit participants were directly engaged in the consultation process. Feedback obtained at the summit was incorporated into the final draft of the roadmap. The final roadmap was endorsed by all Australian states and territories in May 2020.

4. Results

The roadmap is a strategic document [7]. It reflects the reality that the education and training provided to the current and future health workforce must be re-shaped in order to meet the existing and emerging digital requirements, and that a partnership with the education sector is essential. This roadmap is designed to be broad in its application, covering the whole of the health workforce, including all clinical and non-clinical roles. The roadmap consists of:

1.   Principles to enable change;
2.   A three-horizon framework reflecting the maturity levels; and
3.   A digital profile framework articulating the expectations of the many stakeholders in health.

These three main components of the roadmap are explained in the sections below.

4.1. Roadmap Principles for Change

The roadmap starts the process to conceptualise the changes required. Consequently, the key principles of the roadmap are as follows:

- National alignment, collaboration and accountability;
- Flexibility to respond to diverse digital technologies, digital maturity variations and operational environments;
- Leveraging of partnerships to drive innovation;
- Equity of access to healthcare for all Australians, acknowledging the requirement for 'digital inclusion';
- Ethical use of data and information;
- Responsiveness to government and community priorities; and
- Focus on tangible actions and measurable objectives.

4.2. Strategic Horizons Shaping Digital Health

Three horizons explore the workforce and education changes required to support the adoption of digital health technologies.

The horizons will be progressed in parallel, reflecting the different stages of digital health maturity across the health system (see figure 1). There are elements of each of these horizons already visible in the Australian health sector today, and these pockets of innovation need to be shared to provide momentum for positive change, helping Australia harness the digital health opportunities ahead.

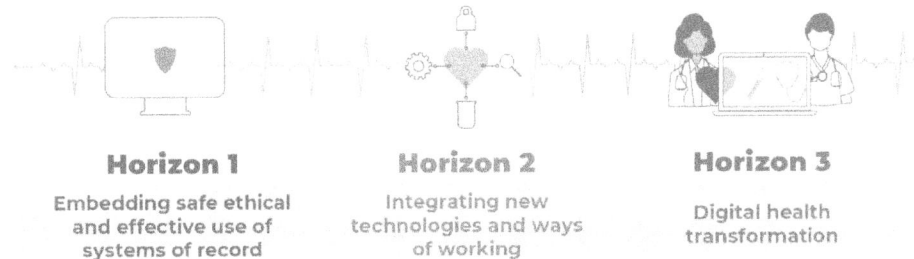

Horizon 1

Embedding safe ethical
and effective use of
systems of record

Horizon 2

Integrating new
technologies and ways
of working

Horizon 3

Digital health
transformation

Figure 1. Horizons based view.

The Horizon 1 vision is for the health workforce and Australian consumers to safely and ethically use digital health tools and to make decisions based on the health information they can access. The Horizon 2 vision is for health systems and organisations to be better connected through interoperability, thereby enabling the health workforce to analyse information, plan and respond to health demands. Emerging digital technologies will reshape health functions and new roles will emerge. The focus will be on enterprise transformation. Finally, the vision of Horizon 3 is that healthcare delivery is transformed through initiatives such as value-based healthcare, personalised medicine, empowered consumers, and care in the home or community, all underpinned by interoperable digital technologies.

Targeted educational interventions are identified within each horizon as follows:

- Horizon 1: Electronic medical record and electronic medication management
- Horizon 2: Artificial intelligence and advanced robotics
- Horizon 3: Personalised medicine, devices, and the integration of the Internet of Things and big data

4.3. Digital Profiles Framework

The purpose of the digital profiles framework is to articulate the expectations of the health workforce as a result of the adoption of digital health technologies. There are eight digital profiles across the health workforce, which include volunteers and healthcare consumers (see figure 2). The framework is designed to provide clarity for key education and health partners who will develop curricula, training and resources to assist the workforce, and to empower health workers and consumers to recognise and grow their digital capability.

The digital profiles identified are applicable in different contexts (including, but not limited to, primary care, aged care, home and community care, and hospitals) and different settings (including in metropolitan, regional, rural and remote locations). While they are designed primarily with a health service delivery focus, health policy and planning roles are also included in the Leadership and Executive, and Business, Administrative and Support Digital Profiles. Given the variety of occupations and qualifications across the health workforce, profiles are not intended to be specific to individual professions. Instead, they are designed to supplement and support the specific knowledge, skills and capabilities of health professions and specialities.

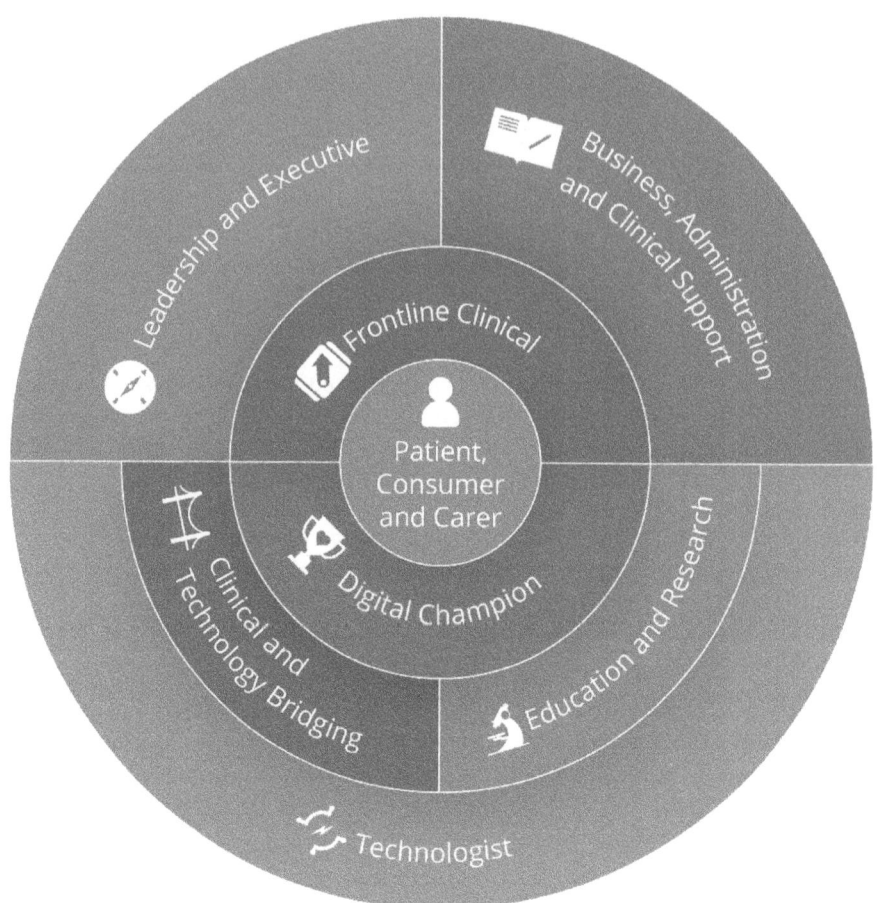

Figure 2. Digital profiles.

The roadmap document [7] articulates in detail the functions of each digital profile and their respective role in contributing to advancing the digital capability of the workforce in health.

5. Next Steps to Implement the Roadmap

In order to support jurisdictions, healthcare organisations, and groups who are identified in the roadmap to implement its recommendations, a Capability Action Plan (CAP) will be developed. The CAP will contemplate, in detail, the roles and responsibilities, timeframes and targets for each stakeholder group across Australia. This will be developed with all partners, including government, universities and education providers, accreditors, and clinical and consumer peaks. This process will ensure the CAP appropriately represents sector priorities, can harmonise the work already occurring both nationally and within jurisdictions, and has funding sources identified. It will also ensure that roles and responsibilities are clear, and organisations support the approach.

It is the critical next step to ensure implementation of the roadmap and realisation of the benefits that will flow to Australia's health workforce.

To complement the mission of the roadmap to support workforce development in digital health, the Australian Digital Health Agency has developed an Emergency Department Clinician's Guide to My Health Record in ED, in collaboration with the Australian Commission on Safety and Quality in Health Care [8]. The agency is also developing the following resources in partnership with clinical peak organisations and technology leaders in these fields:

- National Nursing and Midwifery Digital Health Capability Framework;
- Digital Health Specialist Toolkit;
- Mental Health Resource Compendium; and
- Digital Health Capabilities Framework for the medical profession.

6. Conclusion

The development of the National Digital Health Workforce and Education Roadmap acknowledges that, in Australia, we need to shape how education and training enable our health workforce to realise the benefits of technology, while recognising that people are the health sector's most valuable asset. The roadmap consists of principles, a three-horizon framework reflecting the maturity levels, and a digital profile framework to articulate the expectations of the healthcare stakeholders. A Capability Action Plan is underway to operationalise the key activities proposed in the roadmap.

References

[1]   Australian Digital Health Agency. Australia's National Digital Health Strategy: Safe, Seamless and Secure. Sydney: Australian Government; 2017.
[2]   Shaw T, Hines M, Kielly-Carroll C. Impact of digital health on the safety and quality of health care. Australian Commission on Safety and Quality in Health Care. Sydney: 2017.
[3]   Topol E. The Topol Review: Preparing the Healthcare workforce to deliver the digital future. Health Education England NHS. United Kingdom: 2019.
[4]   Global Digital Health Partnership. Global Digital Health Partnership: 2020, accessed 7/8/20, available from: https://www.gdhp.org/our-vision.
[5]   Brunner M, et al. An eHealth Capabilities Framework for Graduates and Health Professionals: Mixed-Methods Study. J Med Internet Res. 2018; 20(5):e10229.
[6]   Makeham MA, Ryan A. Sharing information safely and securely: the foundation of a modern health care system. The Medical Journal of Australia. 2019; 210(6):S3-S4.
[7]   Australian Digital Health Agency. National Digital Health Workforce and Education Roadmap. Sydney: Australian Government; 2020.
[8]   Australian Commission on Safety and Quality in Health Care. Emergency Department Clinicians' Guide to My Health Record in ED: 2019, accessed 7/8/20, available from: https://www.safetyandquality.gov.au/our-work/e-health-safety/my-health-record-guide.

Healthier Lives, Digitally Enabled
M. Merolli et al. (Eds.)
© 2021 The authors and IOS Press.
This article is published online with Open Access by IOS Press and distributed under the terms
of the Creative Commons Attribution Non-Commercial License 4.0 (CC BY-NC 4.0).
doi:10.3233/SHTI210015

Getting to the Right Patient at the Right Time: An Interoperable Mobile App to Track the ED Journey in Hospital

Audrey P WANG [a,1], David PRYCE [b] and Phillip GOUGH [c]

[a] *The University of Sydney Faculty of Medicine and Health*
[b] *Western Sydney Local Health District*
[c] *The University of Sydney School of Architecture Design and Planning*

Abstract. The current legacy ICT framework structures in healthcare are often siloed and do not allow information to flow easily between business analytics and clinical systems, affecting critical decision making. Western Sydney Local Health District (WSLHD) has numerous electronic database systems for business analytics including tracking individual patients waiting for treatment in the emergency department (ED). Administrators of hospital business data report ED performance measures in a weekly static feedback report to clinical and executive staff due to current legacy systems and manual resource allocation processes. The remit of the project was to prototype a system that could integrate data sources from the current QlikSense Dashboard into an interoperable mobile app with the future intention of direct impact on clinical care decision making for the emergency department. A series of meetings between business analytics unit and clinical staff were used to inform a set of requirements for information workflow systems integration to be used on the project. Stimulated patient data that matched typical data feeds from the system was used to develop a prototype interoperable HL7 messaging mobile app that would report waiting patients in their triage categories in near real time. This working protype with synthetic scenarios and data will inform a future deployable production system with information for the patient journey from the ED waiting room into available hospital beds. As most applications are either designed for business analytics or clinical workflows, integrating information data sources into one mobile application that could meet the needs of both clinical and business performance was novel and integral. This proof of concept project successfully integrated the information systems necessary for both purposes and informs future requirements for an interoperable and deployable cross-platform mobile app.

Keywords. interoperability, mobile applications, triage, HL7, emergency department

1. Introduction

Timely information in the emergency department (ED) allows oversight of: how many people are waiting; level of critical patients in triage categories; and availability of beds in different hospitals. This assists in managing fluctuating surges in demand and supply of emergency services. An example of this is a website that publishes NSW hospital

---

[1] Corresponding Author, Dr. Audrey P Wang, Discipline of Biomedical Informatics and Digital Health, School of Medical Sciences, Faculty of Medicine and Health, The University of Sydney. E-mail: Audrey.wang1@sydney.edu.au.

emergency department waiting times to allow the general public an overview of the number of patients assessed by a triage nurse and waiting for treatment at their local hospital. The simplified overview includes how many patients are waiting over a three-hour period from historical data and the general number of beds/treatment spaces in the Emergency Department [1]. Although the information is periodically refreshed throughout the day approximately every 20 minutes; it remains far from real-time.

Metrics from routinely collected hospital data are often siloed in legacy IT systems making it difficult to provide timely insights for frontline clinicians. The local provision of timely information at emergency departments on similar metrics for key ED clinical decision makers could improve feedback loops for resource allocations closer to the real-time pressures experienced. Candidate metrics include waiting times, triage categories and availability of hospital beds in wards for admission post arrivals at the emergency department. These key metrics are usually collected for two different purposes in a busy metropolitan Sydney hospital: first for business analytics of hospital performance and for operational reporting to centrally based NSW Health systems.

The business analytics department and emergency department identified the need for a redesigned data analytics application that is accessible on mobile devices, interoperable, and applicable for clinicians' provision of patient care. The current application is used across the WSLHD's four hospitals to measure key performance indicators (KPI) of the emergency department performance. The KPIs are built from patient and operations data that helps the ED measure how efficiently resources are used and effectiveness of patient care. The current application is powered by Qlik Sense, a proprietary business software tool not easily accessible, nor interoperable on different platforms. We hypothesised it would be ideal to implement an interoperable mobile application for data analytics, for both WSLHD clinicians and business analysts to resolve the timeliness of critical data metrics mentioned to ensure smooth transition of care across multiple settings.

2. Requirements for WSLHD ED Interoperable Mobile App

The WSLHD emergency department required a redesigned data analytics application which is accessible on cross-platform mobile, interoperable, and more useful for clinicians' provision of patient care. The current web-based application is used across the WSLHD's four hospitals to measure KPIs of the emergency department. The KPIs are built from patient and operations data which help the ED measure how efficiently resources are used and how effectively patients are cared for. Overall, the outcome will be a data analytics application available on smartphones which is interoperable and useful for both WSLHD clinicians and business analysts.

2.1. Background to Existing Systems

The current, non-interoperable, Qlik Sense business application is not part of current clinical workflows and exists as a dashboard on an internal web portal. Clinician's current workflow requires access to numbers of patients waiting in triage, their categories and bed flow management from the patient portal. It provides frontline staff with managerial responsibilities in the emergency department information in an easy to use modality via a mobile phone.

We received a set of requirements following a series of internal inter-departmental meetings. These included developing a conceptual working mobile application (mApp) protype with a new design and framework that would have operationally timely information request systems and updates (< 5 minutes) once deployed with all 32 metrics from the Qlik Sense dashboard in the new cross-platform mobile app. The display would be a clean and user-friendly visualisation, allowing clinicians to access any metrics within 10 seconds of launching the application. It also must have no real patient or hospital data latently stored on the device to ensure the privacy and security of sensitive data. The users would use familiar data security and privacy authentication systems. The mApp should be interoperable and identify capabilities for SMART on FHIR standards [2, 3] and have an application programming interface (API) that could be used to support extended functionality including bed management in the future. Finally, information requests and updates must occur in the timely manner for operational usefulness when deployed.

The mApp includes the following functional requirements: First, users will be able to securely login to the application using their work credentials. Data will be displayed for one hospital location at a time and allow for easy navigation to other locations. Each location will be displayed in a similar format to allow for comparison. Finally, the application will provide additional information on demand about the data being displayed, so users are able to understand the information, following W3C protocols to ensure the app has high usability for a wide base of users (e.g. hearing or vision impaired).

3. Prototype Overview

The prototype included a front end, back end consisting of an interoperable Python Flask framework with interactions into the backend database, with existing HL7 [4] standards server populated with mock patient data, called with HL7 messaging APIs. The current QlikSense web-based application receives data from an existing PostgresSQL database continuously updated from a wide range of legacy IT systems that contain patient related emergency department data. The data includes how long the person has been waiting post front-desk administration registration and the number of patients allocated to each triage category. A diagram of the structure for System Integration implementation is provided in Figure 1.

The mApp prototype system's cross-platform front end was built using the JavaScript-based React Native framework. Other dependencies included Node.js and Expo. The Expo Client App allowed live testing of the application on any mobile phone and can be downloaded from Apple App Store or Google Play Store for Android. A Flask server microframework was implemented to support the functional requirements and create the system's middle API, built using Python code. It has modular dependencies that can be interoperable. The middle API utilised the SQL Alchemy Python module to interact with the dummy version of the database used by the hospital, built using PostgreSQL. Further dependencies for developing a functional API include Flask-Script, Flask-Migrate, Psycopg2 and APScheduler.

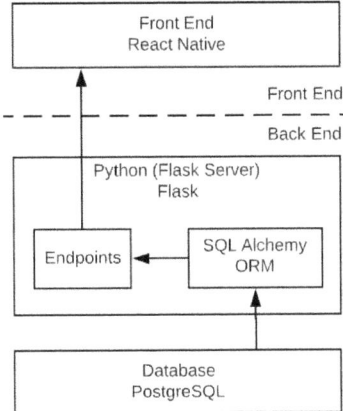

Figure 1. High level architecture diagram of mApp prototype.

4. Testing Results

The development team utilised various tests and tools to verify and validate system integration functionalities. The feedback findings from inter-departmental meetings were heavily relied upon to test the front-end prototype functionalities. A range of tests were instigated to determine if the mApp could be successfully deployed in the future base on the current system integration framework profile:

Unit Tests - Automated tests to check the output for the smaller modules of the program. This has been automated. For the backend, the tests done were to check if the API correctly includes all the ED KPIs for the react code to fetch data from. The frontend tests here were mainly done to establish if the rendered screen exists and comparing them to the snapshots of the determined wireframes.

Integration Tests - Testing the connection to the database.

Functional Tests - Manual tests to check whether system responds correctly according to the different predetermined functions.

The test coverage of the codebase is achieved across three testing areas: the front-end testing of the React Native codebase, back-end testing of the Python codebase, and durability stress testing of the system. The dummy database itself does not need to be tested because the codebase has been provided by WSLHD. The app was tested and able to sustain 100 users simultaneously and was pressured tested to 1000 concurrent pulls on the server for 10 seconds using apache Benchmark. The response rate was 3.5 seconds. Consideration of the code base adherence to SMART on FHIR standards were considered in the project. All changes conforming to HL7 message standards were already in place (from the hospital team prior to this project) for database informatics pulls. All other code base adhered to open source concepts using python language and any API standards used could be modified for REST API standards.

Automated test coverage was 60% for the front end. The rest of the coverage were tested using manual testing. This included testing the app's functional output to deliver login authentication, correct page navigation and appropriate key performance indicator data items. Login in credentials mimic NSW Health methods for authentication tested well in the prototype between the database and login screen. This performed well as a necessary gateway into the app. The application will need integration into the NSW

Health authentication and encryption system during live deployment in the future. Automation of user log out occurs if static use of one page is for more than 5 minutes. Automated testing is shown in Table 1. The stress test is for the cross-platform application when hosted on a local machine allowed a transfer rate of 628.60 Kbytes/sec. As a result, the stress test is largely testing the speed and robustness of the network interactions and system structure. The stress test must be repeated once deployed to a real environment where the system is connected to WSLHD servers. There was no latent cache of data required and therefore allows protection of sensitive patient related data once user logged out.

Table 1. Automated testing results.

Test	Codebase tested	Type	Result
Front end coverage	React Native	Automated	60%
Back end coverage	Python (Flask)	Automated	87%
Durability and stress testing	System	Automated	mean: 3.7s, max: 3.8s, min: 0.062s

4.1. Limitations

We identified four live-deployment limitations. First, authentication systems were not live tested for NSW Health authentication systems, but the prototype allows for the necessary security protocols to be embedded into the app. Also, validation of HL7 messages will need to have a framework of testing that will ensure quality control of messaging to draw the data from a much larger live regularly updated database. Further, the mock prototype app which is functional and able to call up synthetic aggregated patient data could have extended functionality to individual patient data. Finally, we have a placeholder for patient flow portal services to assist with database updates for beds for WSLHD. This functionality was not prototyped fully due to limited time and stakeholder availability for this function during the period of the project. We also identified one limitation through pressure testing. The Flask server has the ability to integrate more interoperable extensions including Flask-RESTful for building REST APIs or proxy servers, that will allow further adherence to SMART on FHIR standards. This will be part of the proposed development for future deployment.

5. Discussion and Conclusion

Overall, the prototype of across-platform mobile application for Emergency Department data was determined to be largely be a success. The working data analytics network connections were prototyped as useful for both hospital clinicians and business analysts to resolve the timeliness of critical data metrics to ensure smooth transition of care across multiple settings. The success was measured by having a reproducible working code base with documentation that resulted in a final deployable cross-platform mobile app. Sample aggregated patient data could be displayed and lower level data breakdown to individual patient data could be extended for live deployment. The data in the application updates within five-minute intervals or less, as demonstrated by the pressure tests, from the dummy database. The privacy of patient and hospital data was secure by ensuring data is never saved to the individual device. A higher level of authentication protocol could be implemented in the future where the usernames match the current NSW Health systems.

This project had time and scope limitations for project completion. Therefore, product success criterion that were not achievable in this iteration included:

- The application can be successfully uploaded onto a cross-platform phone by anyone.
- The data in the application is read from the WSLHD database directly.
- The application can connect to WSLHD databases offsite.
- Successful in vivo usability tests conducted with actual clinicians to assess the value of data analytics tool.
- The presence of an initial application directory page for additional extensions.

Overall, the system structure served well for the development where the application was kept local to the machine and isolated from the WSLHD servers, using a middle network of APIs. Upon real deployment onto the ED floor using WSLHD databases, a different set of network interactions involving a server proxy is likely to be required if data accessibility issues arise. Future work will be needed to address the limitations of the current interoperable mobile app for live deployment to ensure all implementation success criterion are met. In conclusion, we achieved adequate evidence to support our hypothesis of the required integration of siloed systems to demonstrate success in integration of clinical and business analytics to track the patient journey in ED.

Acknowledgements

We would like to acknowledge the contributions of Katherine Sutarlim, Abhinandan Srinivas, Onam Khan, Antonia Mijatovic, Dugald Shannon in working on the prototype as part of a capstone student software group project. Adhish Panta, Jim Cook and Viji Venkataramani as part of the collaboration with the ICT Tech Lab and School of Computer Science, University of Sydney. Reshma Kolambkar for providing HL7 expertise and codebase, and Margaret Murphy for her clinical emergency department expertise, to build the necessary system interactions into clinically relevant workflows. A demonstration of the app was given in the University of Sydney Westmead Innovation Showcase. Institutional ethical approval was given WSLHD HREC QA2009-16.

References

[1]   Health N. Emergency Department waiting times in major NSW hospitals 2020 [Accessed 14/02/2020]. Available from: https://www.emergencywait.health.nsw.gov.au/#a.
[2]   Mandel JC, Kreda DA, Mandl KD, Kohane IS, Ramoni RB. SMART on FHIR: a standards-based, interoperable apps platform for electronic health records. Journal of the American Medical Informatics Association. 2016;23(5):899-908.
[3]   Metke-Jimenez A, Harrap K, Conlan D, Gibson S, Pearson J, Hansen D, editors. A SMART on FHIR Prototype for Genomic Test Ordering. Digital Health: Changing the Way Healthcare is Conceptualised and Delivered: Selected Papers from the 27th Australian National Health Informatics Conference (HIC 2019); 2019: IOS Press.
[4]   Lopez DM, Blobel B. Architectural approaches for HL7-based health information systems implementation. Methods of information in medicine. 2010;49(2):196-204.

Healthier Lives, Digitally Enabled
M. Merolli et al. (Eds.)
© 2021 The authors and IOS Press.
This article is published online with Open Access by IOS Press and distributed under the terms
of the Creative Commons Attribution Non-Commercial License 4.0 (CC BY-NC 4.0).
doi:10.3233/SHTI210016

Visual Design and Anthropomorphism in a Mobile Pulmonary Rehabilitation Support Intervention

Cindy CHONG [a], Danielle LOTTRIDGE [a], Jim WARREN [a,1] and Rosie DOBSON [b]
a School of Computer Science, University of Auckland
b National Institute for Health Innovation, University of Auckland

Abstract. Pulmonary rehabilitation is a behavioral intervention that can improve symptom control and quality of life for patients with chronic obstructive pulmonary disease (COPD), but access, uptake and adherence are problematic. Our team has pursued the development of a mobile phone-based intervention (mobile pulmonary rehabilitation, mPR) with iterative design and a pilot study. The mPR intervention is delivered through two technologies: text messages (SMS) and a smartphone application. Our user-centered design analysis of pilot study data led to several insights. First, patients' replies to the SMS suggested that messages were anthropomorphised and provided social support. Second, the smartphone application could help patients by clearly visualizing the exercise program, alternative exercises, and progress to date. We demonstrate the design iterations made to meet these requirements and we present feedback obtained from experts and from four COPD patients. We discuss implications for the design of mobile pulmonary rehabilitation interventions.

Keywords. mobile applications, consumer health informatics, chronic disease management, human-computer interaction, user experience, mHealth

1. Introduction

One of the gold standard interventions for the ongoing management of chronic obstructive pulmonary disease (COPD) is pulmonary rehabilitation (PR) which comprises of a supervised, individually tailored, multidisciplinary program of exercise training, breathing retraining and improving patient knowledge through education. A systematic review of participation in physical activity programs, including PR, identified barriers including changing health status and lack of support and enablers including specific goals and social and professional support [1].

To increase the reach of pulmonary rehabilitation, the development of a mobile based intervention (mobile pulmonary rehabilitation, mPR) has been pursued via a project initiated in mid-2018. Modern mobile devices ('smartphones') support multiple distinct modalities for interventions. The capability of text message (SMS) programs to promote healthy behaviors with personalised interventions is well established and includes smoking cessation [2] as well as concurrent reduction in multiple cardiac risk

---

[1] Corresponding Author, Jim Warren, School of Computer Science, University of Auckland, Auckland 1142, New Zealand; E-mail: jim@cs.auckland.ac.nz.

factors for patients with coronary heart disease [3]. Health promoting apps can include images and video, collect feedback with sensors (from the phone or other devices), provide graphical feedback on progress and support diaries [4, 5]. Health promoting interventions using mobile technology can facilitate rehabilitation in a variety of straightforward ways: through reminders and provision of easily accessible informational resources such exercises based on individual health status. Decades of experimental social science indicates that in many circumstances, people relate to computers in essentially social ways similar to the ways they relate to other people [6] (*aka* anthropomorphizing the system) As such, we suggest that mobile interventions can also offer something that might be unexpected from a technology: social support.

In this paper we present work on improving the user experience of the app component of a combined SMS and app based mPR intervention, based on identifying complementary roles of the SMS and app channels.

2. Original mPR Design, Intervention and Pilot Field Test

A mixed-methods (survey and interview) study undertaken for this project found high interest in mPR from both patients and healthcare professionals [7]. While participants saw the potential to improve access to PR through technology, there was concern about access to technology and digital literacy, as well as patient safety and the lack of group environment (as compared to gold standard PR). Patients and healthcare professionals identified key features for a mPR intervention, leading to the development of an mPR intervention with both personalised and tailored SMS and mobile app components.

The SMS intervention spanned 9 weeks; one core message per day provided motivation, support and information. There was also a weekly SMS exercise prescription message (at one of three baseline exercise capacity levels as defined by the enrolling PR clinician), smoking cessation support for smokers, and a weekly message on airway clearance for those with high secretion load. There was an optional family/ whānau version of the messages for those supporting the patient. Messages were personalised and tailored with the person's name, culturally specific greeting and names of any support people that were added. Example SMS messages include:

- Motivation: "mPR: [hi]. By doing the mPR program you can improve balance, muscle strength, general fitness, & general wellbeing. We are here to support you!"
- Support: "mPR: [hi] [name]. If there is something concerning you or your family about your health it's a good idea to discuss it with your doctor or nurse"
- Exercise information: "mPR: It is normal to feel a bit stiff after you first start to exercise as your muscles may not be used to the exercises. Keep going - the stiffness will ease"

The mPR app was an optional addition to the SMS. The app provided goal-setting, videos of people completing the prescribed exercises at the patient's baseline exercise capacity, self-assessments (questionnaire and 1-minute sit to stand test), and reminders. The app also included relaxation audio files and information for family for their support role. Figure 1 shows a selection of screens.

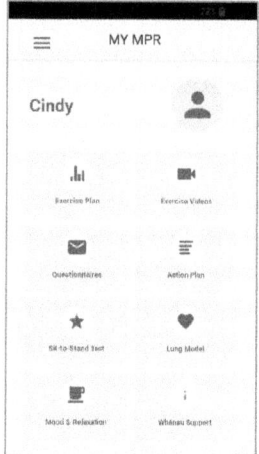 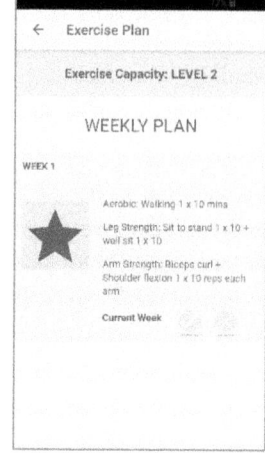 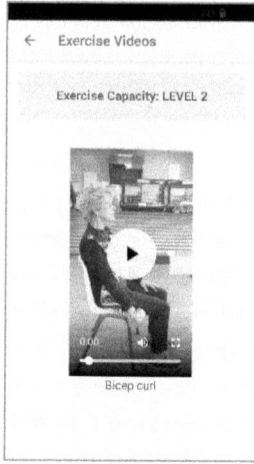

Figure 1. Screenshots of the initial mPR app that was deployed in the pilot study: (a) Dashboard screen; (b) Exercise Plan screen (c) Exercise Video screen.

A non-randomised pilot study of mPR was conducted between July and November 2019; 26 people with chronic respiratory disease who were eligible for PR participated, as well as 4 family members of participants. 18 participants (70%) opted to use the app as well as SMS; of those, 11 signed-in to the app. 20 were available for follow-up interviews of whom 19 (95%) said mPR helped them feel more supported, and 17 (85%) said it helped them change their behavior. Full results are published elsewhere [8].

Of the 26 participants, 23 sent 390 SMS replies including exercise counts, health ratings, STOP messages, feedback messages and unexpected messages. Unexpected messages included updates: "Yup I do that and go shopping walking around supermarket" and "I am probably going to have a difficult time doing everything this week as in my car a lot!!" They asked questions such as "When I go home are you ok with me doing one walk in the water [pool] as causes no problems. Thanks." They made other remarkable responses: "[these messages are] what I've been looking for ages." and "Thank you for the support over the mPR program and thanks to all involved". There were 109 unexpected messages sent by 17 participants; 40 were Thank you messages, 11 were "Ok" and 6 were emoji message (sent from the same participant). The apparent anthropomorphizing of the SMS agent led us to note that SMS could act as social support to some participants, in addition to providing reminders and high-level information.

When patients were asked what they found most useful on the app, the most frequent response was the exercise videos. This was corroborated by examining the usage logs: exercise videos were viewed 88 times. When asked for suggestions of how the app could be improved, several patients mentioned they wanted to see their individual progress. Patients' feedback also led to requirements to add greater variability in exercises and simplify navigation. We noted that eight subsections of the application were given equal priority via equal screen real estate on the dashboard screen. In order to visually emphasise the most important functionality, we re-assigned screen space to functions that were most crucial and frequently accessed.

3. App Re-design

We used a user-centered design approach [9] to reconsider app design requirements from subject matter experts, patients, and usage logs. We analyzed the functions delivered by the SMS intervention to determine requirements for the smartphone app. Together with the team, we confirmed that the highest priority of the smartphone app was to support access to information about the exercise program. Thus, the main needs for the app "home screen" would be high-level and related to the exercise program. Given the patients' user needs, design priorities, and the support provided through SMS, we designed a presentation of progress through the exercise program that could be holistically scanned "at a glance", i.e., glanceable. High-fidelity prototypes were created and shown to PR and m-Health experts for feedback. Comments were collated and edits were made to the prototype before re-showing the PR and m-Health experts to confirm the decisions in the re-design.

The re-design focused on three major areas: the home page, the exercise prescription page, and the videos page (Figure 2). No components of the app were removed. Components that were not prioritised were accessible from the menu. The prioritised focus of the app is exercise, which is why this component takes up approximately 80% of the home screen real estate (Figure 2a). The main screen has circles that fill in to represent progress towards completion of daily activity targets. There is a greyscale path through the exercises to provide patients with recommended ordering. The grey path was intentionally subtle to not divert visual emphasis from the exercises. Below the menu is a personalised welcome message to promote a feeling of personalisation. The bottom component of the main screen was prioritised for the other identified key elements that support COPD patients: breathing exercises, completion charts ("My progress") and what to do if feeling unwell. The menu on the top left includes the functions that were less used in the pilot study or were determined as not critical to the main functionality and focus of the app. These were self-assessment questionnaires, lung video, help documentation. Each exercise page included alternatives for the recommended exercise and accompanying videos (Figure 2b, 2c). When selected, the exercise videos open to a larger screen for easier viewing (Figure 2c). The green checkmark and green around the exercise icons indicates the patient's progress per day for each exercise (Figure 2a, 2b).

4. Testing

To evaluate the usability of the redesigned prototype, we sought feedback from clinicians and patients with usability testing methodology from user-centered design [9]. There were 4 patients, a nurse, a physiotherapist, and a doctor who agreed to take part. Two of the patients participated in the pilot study and so had familiarity with the earlier version of the app. User testing consisted of individual face to face sessions looking at a clickable prototype on a mobile phone, which was first demonstrated by the researcher and then handed over to the participant. A semi-structured interview format prompted discussion with asking about what was useful/liked and not useful/disliked and what other functions might be wanted. All participants were able to discover and view all parts of the app. Two out of four patients were positive about the app's overall usability with the comments the app "seemed easy to use" and "it looks like something I would use"; one was positive about components of the app and the fourth was neutral.

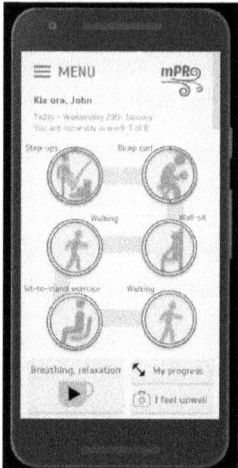 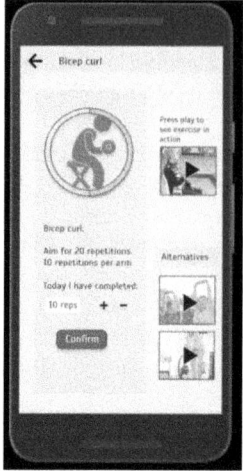 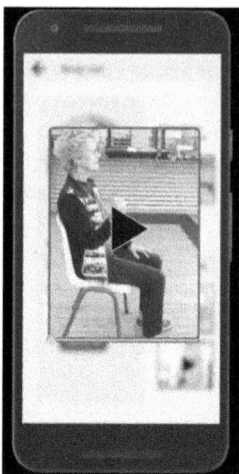

Figure 2. Screenshots of the re-designed mPR app based on design insights from the pilot study: (a) Home screen; (b) An exercise prescription screen; (c) Bicep curl video screen.

The exercise prescription and progress screens were well received. One patient stated: "This looks really good though, it looks like something I would use". Another stated: "Lets you know if you're slacking off sometimes, or maybe not going as well as you should for whatever reason." In Figure 2b, the grey path was intended to be a path which patients could follow to do exercises in a prescribed order; however, patients did not explore the exercises in this order. One of the clinicians did not understand the meaning of the path and thought it was "decoration," indicating the need to clarify further what is the 'next' exercise to be completed. No patient asked for clarification about the green progress circles, but one of the clinicians asked for clarification on them, indicating they may not be sufficiently emphasised or intuitive. The feedback received resulted in minor design revisions. We plan to use this redesign in an upcoming field trial.

5. Discussion and Conclusion

User-centered design and analysis applied to a mPR intervention resulted in insights related to complementary roles of the intervention's SMS and smartphone app technologies. The insights and user feedback led to substantial redesign of the app. The most notable aspect of the re-design was a glanceable presentation of the exercise program that incorporated progress. The main page of the re-designed app also prioritised other crucial features for COPD patients: e.g. what to do if acutely unwell. This approach is in line with Tendedez et al. [10] who found that patients with chronic respiratory conditions tended to use technology to manage their conditions reactively, such as recording peak flow readings or using their healthcare apps when they were feeling poorly and stopping self-managing or monitoring when they felt well.

In terms of future work, anthropomorphizing of the SMS was an insight from the user-centered design analysis; the strength of the social relationships and potential benefits or risks should be investigated. Further, there is potential for wearable technology and mobile sensors to track physical activity which would reduce patients' recording burden. Such monitoring technologies were not integrated with this app but will be investigated in future work. There are still basic barriers to use for smartphone apps; users had difficulties logging into the app. We encourage extensive evaluation testing of login to ensure this is not a barrier to use. More broadly, issues related to the relative isolation of patients when doing mPR, such as safety in doing exercises as well as loss of social interaction, are an ongoing consideration. The most recent round of testing has obvious limitations of small sample size and limited user exposure to the app.

The combination of SMS-based interventions and a smartphone app is potentially powerful for delivering behavioral interventions such as pulmonary rehabilitation. SMS is more accessible due to simplicity of user interaction and, even in 2020, due to technical ubiquity (e.g. not everybody has a data plan even if they have a smartphone). However, smartphones offer features, such as providing videos and graphical feedback on progress, that can meaningfully expand the user experience of the intervention. This work has highlighted the value in understanding the relationship of these two mobile phone based modalities to guide app design, suggesting a surprisingly social role for SMS and a complementary informational, visual and progress-tracking roles for the smartphone app.

Acknowledgements

This work was funded by a Medtech CoRE grant. We thank the participants of the mPR pilot study, and the patients and clinicians at the pulmonary rehabilitation programs for their invaluable feedback. Thanks to Manoj Alwis for his feedback on design and implementation. Thanks to the mPR co-investigators and particularly Julie Reeve, Gayl Humphrey and Sarah Candy for their feedback on this manuscript.

References

[1] O. Thorpe, K. Johnston, and S. Kumar, "Barriers and enablers to physical activity participation in patients with COPD: a systematic review," *J Cardiopulm Rehabil Prev,* vol. 32, no. 6, pp. 359-69, Nov-Dec 2012.

[2] R. Whittaker, H. McRobbie, C. Bullen, A. Rodgers, Y. Gu, and R. Dobson, "Mobile phone text messaging and app-based interventions for smoking cessation," *Cochrane Database Syst Rev,* vol. 10, p. CD006611, Oct 22 2019.

[3] C. K. Chow *et al.,* "Effect of Lifestyle-Focused Text Messaging on Risk Factor Modification in Patients With Coronary Heart Disease: A Randomized Clinical Trial," *JAMA,* vol. 314, no. 12, pp. 1255-63, Sep 22-29 2015.

[4] J. P. Higgins, "Smartphone Applications for Patients' Health and Fitness," *Am J Med,* vol. 129, no. 1, pp. 11-9, Jan 2016.

[5] K. L. Barnes, G. Dunivan, A. Jaramillo-Huff, T. Krantz, J. Thompson, and P. Jeppson, "Evaluation of Smartphone Pelvic Floor Exercise Applications Using Standardized Scoring System," *Female Pelvic Med Reconstr Surg,* vol. 25, no. 4, pp. 328-335, Jul/Aug 2019.

[6] B. Reeves and C. Nass, *The media equation: How people treat computers, television, and new media like real people and places.* Center for Study of Language and Information; Cambridge University Press, 1996.

[7] R. Dobson *et al.,* "Understanding End-User Perspectives of Mobile Pulmonary Rehabilitation (mPR): Cross-Sectional Survey and Interviews," *JMIR Form Res,* vol. 3, no. 4, p. e15466, Dec 20 2019.

[8] R. Whittaker *et al.,* "Mobile Pulmonary Rehabilitation (mPR): Pilot Study of a Prototype Mobile Phone-based Program," *Frontiers in Computer Science,* vol. under review, 2020.

[9] J. Preece, H. Sharp, and Y. Rogers, *Interaction Design: Beyond Human-Computer Interaction,* 4th ed. Wiley, 2015.

[10] H. Tendedez, M. Ferrario, and R. McNaney, "Respiratory self-care: Identifying current challenges and future potentials for digital technology to support people with chronic respiratory conditions," in *Proceedings of the 13th EAI International Conference on Pervasive Computing Technologies for Healthcare*, 2019, pp. 129-138.

Healthier Lives, Digitally Enabled
M. Merolli et al. (Eds.)
doi:10.3233/SHTI210017

A Chatbot Architecture for Promoting Youth Resilience

Chester HOLT-QUICK [a,b], Jim WARREN [a,1], Karolina STASIAK [b],
Ruth WILLIAMS [b], Grant CHRISTIE [b], Sarah HETRICK [b],
Sarah HOPKINS [b], Tania CARGO [b] and Sally MERRY [b]

[a] *School of Computer Science, University of Auckland*
[b] *Department of Psychological Medicine, University of Auckland*

Abstract. E-health technologies have potential to provide scalable and accessible interventions for youth mental health. As part of an ecosystem of e-screening and e-therapy tools for New Zealand young people, a dialog agent, Headstrong, has been designed to promote resilience with methods grounded in cognitive behavioral therapy and positive psychology. This paper describes the architecture underlying the chatbot. The architecture supports a range of over 20 activities delivered in a 4-week program by relatable personas. The architecture provides a visual authoring interface to its content management system. In addition to supporting the original adolescent resilience chatbot, the architecture has been reused to create a 3-week 'stress-detox' intervention for undergraduates, and subsequently for a chatbot to support young people with the impacts of the COVID-19 pandemic, with all three systems having been used in field trials. The Headstrong architecture illustrates the feasibility of creating a domain-focused authoring environment in the context of e-therapy that supports non-technical expert input and rapid deployment.

Keywords. mobile applications, consumer health informatics, mental health, software engineering

1. Introduction

While most young people in New Zealand report good overall wellbeing, emotional difficulties are prevalent, with young people reporting high levels of depressive symptoms, self-harming behavior and suicidal ideation [1]. Most mental health disorders have an onset in adolescence, a time associated with poor help-seeking and access to services [2], setting the scene for longer-term negative outcomes such as adverse mental health and economic outcomes in early adulthood [3]. A majority of school principals reported being frustrated they could not get help for students with mental health issues, and students in lower socio-economic areas were in greater need of support [4].

Providing e-Health interventions has shown to lead to improved emotional well-being in general [5] and in school settings [6]. E-Health interventions can provide near-universal reach and access, and potentially appeal to young people concerned about the stigma of using the conventional mental health system. Dialog agent or 'chatbot' style

---

[1] Corresponding Author, Jim Warren, School of Computer Science, University of Auckland, Auckland 1142, New Zealand; E-mail: jim@cs.auckland.ac.nz.

interaction for digital mental health has attracted interest since Eliza in the 1960s and evidence of effectiveness has been demonstrated for the modern system, Woebot [7].

The Health Advances through Behavioural Intervention Technologies (HABITs) project has developed an ecosystem of screening and e-therapy tools designed to meet the needs of New Zealand young people with a co-design approach emphasising input from Māori and Pacific youth. The objective is to deliver evidence-based therapy in a form that resonates with local young people. As part of HABITs a chatbot providing dialog-based intervention grounded in cognitive behavioral therapy and positive psychology, called Headstrong, was developed. This paper presents the architecture underlying the Headstrong chatbot, and related chatbots.

2. Conceptual Design of a Chatbot for Resilient Youth

RUSH Digital were selected by tender to partner with the university-based team and our community stakeholders to create the chatbot. A hybrid user-centered design / co-design process was used, beginning with scoping interviews of young people and experienced counselors. This was followed by design workshops including young people, counselors, researchers and developers. The resulting design focuses on daily user engagement in key activities over a 4-week intervention program, including relaxation strategies; problem solving techniques; recognising and tackling negative thoughts; interpersonal and communication skills, using a gratitude journal; and scheduling positive activities.

While Headstrong is fundamentally text dialog based, avatars were designed (see figure 1) to make the chat agent relatable. The avatars are rendered as young people slightly older and more experienced than the intended users, and giving a choice of gender and ethnicity representative of the target population. These avatars appear in various poses during the chat, such as providing a 'selfie' when initially building rapport with the user and with various expressions as appropriate to the messages in the activities.

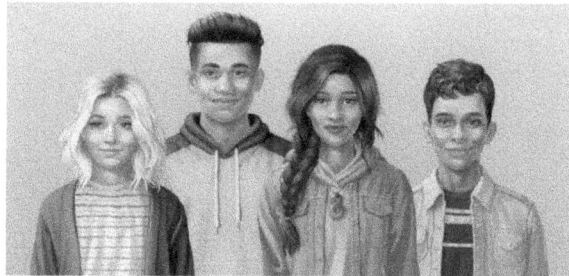

Figure 1. The four Headstrong avatars - from left: Olivia, Manaia, Aroha and Ravi.

3. Headstrong Architecture

Google's Dialogflow (https://dialogflow.com/) and other similar technologies such as Watson Assistant by IBM (https://www.ibm.com/cloud/watson-assistant/) offer simple off-the-shelf solutions to configure and deploy a chatbot and are becoming widely used. Such solutions are well suited to limited question-answering type help chatbots often employed in businesses, but configuring and managing (and visualising) large amounts of content quickly becomes untenable. Implementing the Headstrong design required dialog for more than 20 distinct activities each of which engages users for 5-10 minutes. Further, to streamline knowledge engineering, and provide ease of adaptation for differing audiences and uses, authoring of dialog content should be possible by users without technical expertise. Enhanced functionality was wanted within the conversational channel such as media or minigames; and for research requirements, detailed but ethical tracking of chatbot usage was needed.

Figure 2 illustrates the Headstrong architecture. Facebook Messenger was selected as the front-end to engage young people with a familiar interface likely to be already installed on their phones. The Headstrong server leverages existing components RUSH Digital had deployed to other industries, and uses Dialogflow for matching user input to intents. It interfaces to the HABITs digital platform [8] to record usage data for research. The browser-based interface for dialog authoring is described in the next section.

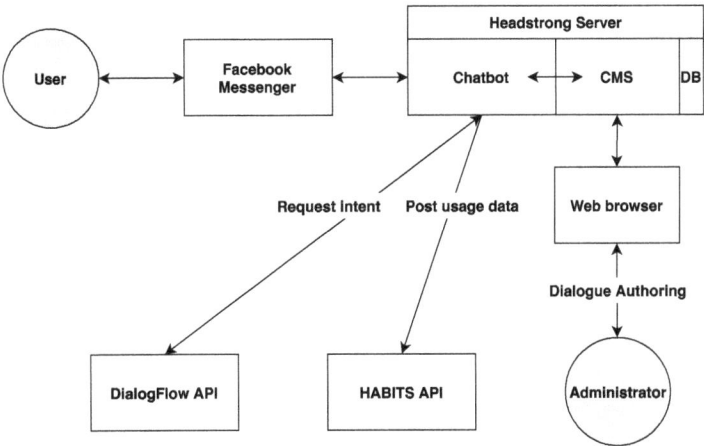

Figure 2. Components of the Headstrong architecture.

4. Content Management and Authoring

To give domain experts the ability to directly author content, a graphical user interface is provided that creates a directed graph structure. Node types are color-coded and dragged down from a toolbar into a working canvas. For example, Figure 3 includes a condition-checking node (pink), with conditions along each branch (beige), a question node (green) with quick reply options (beige) and two modules (lime). The '+' icon on the lower-right of nodes can be clicked to add conditions or options. The resulting graph is a logical flow diagram, intuitive to non-technical users.

There remain aspects of dialog authoring that are too challenging for non-technical users, including configuring the chatbot introduction based on whether the chatbot is responding to unprompted user engagement versus handling response from chatbot-prompted engagement; and reference to prior user state, such as whether the user had expressed distress and triggered the emergency escalation module during the prior engagement. This requires defining and managing user variables and setting up conditional branches to a degree that is beyond the purview of a non-technical user.

Psychologists and other mental health specialists principally authored the activity modules. These consist predominantly of statement nodes (where text is output), questions with quick replies and output media files (e.g., images and animated GIFs).

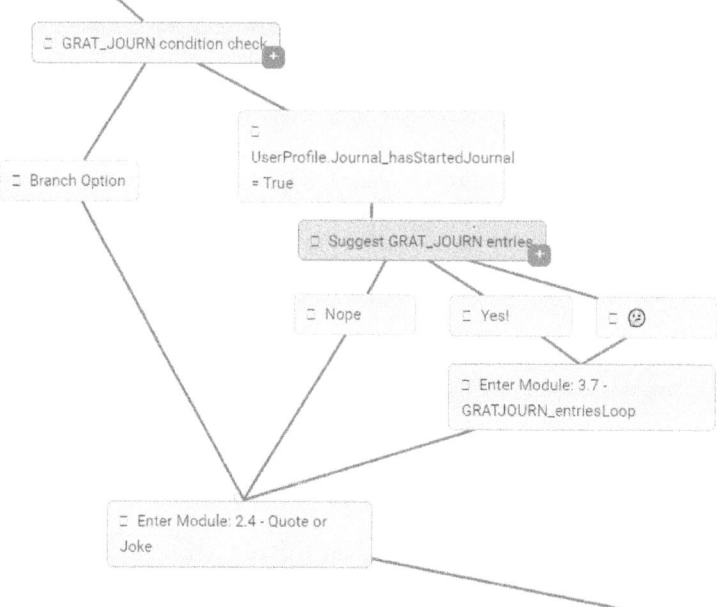

Figure 3. A portion of the daily loop routine as shown on the working canvas.

5. Use and Re-use of the Dialog Architecture

Figure 4 illustrates a snippet of a dialog session as it appears to the end user. After a period of iterative refinement based on feedback from both experts and young people, a field trial was set up using online consent in the HABITs portal. In late 2019, users were recruited from two local secondary schools. While the trial results are outside of the scope of this paper, it can be said that there were no issues from a technical perspective.

Even before the Headstrong field trial commenced, the architecture was re-used for a chatbot called "21-Day Stress Detox" (SD), developed as a Masters research project [9] to foster stress resilience in university undergraduates. Technical features of the architecture aided reuse: (a) a dialog duplication function allows content to be copied, altered and re-used for deployment as another chatbot; (b) it supports deployment of multiple chatbots with distinct dialog, connected to distinct channels (i.e. different Facebook pages) from one running server instance. The SD content was designed for users to engage with the chatbot once per day. Each day the chatbot checks in with the user at a chosen time, asks them to rate their stress level, and begins a new activity module; the day ends with choice of motivational quote, joke or gratitude journal entry. Activity modules are unique each day while other 'daily loop' components are re-used (e.g., introductions are drawn randomly from a pre-authored set). The chatbot was field tested with over 120 undergraduates recruited from several large classes.

A moderate amount of dialog content from Headstrong was able to be reused for SD with minor modification tailored to difference in target age group. Specifically, modules for greeting and farewell, minigames, jokes, meditation, gratitude journaling and risk phrase management were all reused; as was the Dialogflow intent classifier. Reused content constituted roughly half of SD. The novel dialog content was almost completely authored by the psychology Masters student in under 2 months. An initial 2-hour teaching session by a software developer was required, followed by two further sessions to build on the first session and troubleshoot issues. The developer set up the overall logical architecture for the program including management of user variables and resolving errors. Approximately 30 hours of developer time were required. Minimal developer time was required for authoring the unique daily activities.

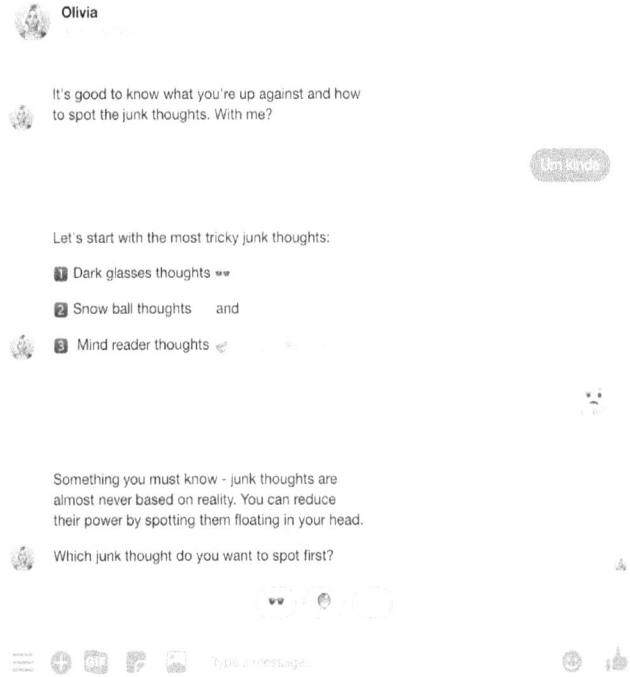

Figure 4. Screen capture of a fragment of Headstrong conversation within one of six cognitive modules targeted at negative thinking.

This set the scene for very rapid development and deployment of Aroha, a chatbot to support young people with impacts related to the COVID-19 pandemic. The overall conversation design was newly created, tailored for expected one-off user-driven engagement with Aroha, differing from the conversation design for Headstrong and SD. Some content (e.g. gratitude journaling, minigames, meditation) from those two projects was re-used through module duplication, with minor modification to the dialog. The main new content for Aroha was developed by two experienced clinical psychologists over one weekend before lockdown in New Zealand. Dialog refinement, testing and implementation of feedback took place over 10 days and then a clinical trial begun.

6. Discussion and Conclusion

An architecture that supports easy authoring and deployment encompassing key requirements of a chatbot to promote resilience in young people has been developed, and has been used for three distinct deployments with different content and audiences. Through the graphical authoring canvas, content creation was largely accomplished by domain experts with technical support required only around areas such as definition of working variables to support branching and reminder logic.

Headstrong dialog is the result of expert adaptation of evidence-based psychological therapies and co-design with target users. Systems like XiaoIce, a social chatbot emphasising emotional connection with over 660 million users [10], show that deep learning can be successfully applied to dialog. Integrating such capabilities (e.g. use of deep-learnt dialog for rapport building and discovery) is a key direction for development with the objective of achieving longer retention in evidence-based programs.

In conclusion, the Headstrong architecture illustrates the feasibility of creating a domain-focused authoring environment for e-therapy. The architecture supports expert input through its visual interface to the content management system. Further, the architecture allows rapid deployment to field studies and sufficient flexibility to support interventions of different lengths and for different target audiences. Work continues to enhance the chatbot's ability to tailor responses for maximum user engagement.

Acknowledgements

The authors thank all the participants in the development process and field trials. The authors have no commercial interest in RUSH Digital but may be designated inventors in Intellectual Property relating to novel dialog components and/or content described in this paper. This work was funded by A Better Start (grant UOAX1511) and CureKids (Discretionary grant 5050).

References

[1]   T. Clark *et al.*, "Health and well-being of secondary school students in New Zealand: Trends between 2001, 2007 and 2012," *Journal of Paediatrics and Child Health,* vol. 49, no. 11, pp. 925-934, 2013.
[2]   N. Reavley, S. Cvetkovski, A. Jorm, and D. Lubman, "Help-seeking for substance use, anxiety and affective disorders among young people: results from the 2007 Australasian National Survey of Mental Health and Wellbeing," *Australian & New Zealand Journal of Psychiatry,* vol. 44, no. 8, pp. 729-735, 2010.
[3]   D. Fergusson, J. M. Boden, and L. J. Horwood, "Recurrence of major depression in adolescence and early adulthood, and later mental health, educational, and economic outcomes," *British Journal of Psychiatry,* vol. 191, pp. 335-342, 2007.
[4]   L. Bonne and J. MacDonald, "Secondary schools in 2018: Findings from the NZCER national survey," New Zealand Council for Educational Research, Wellington, 2019.
[5]   D. D. Ebert *et al.*, "Internet and computer-based cognitive behavioral therapy for anxiety and depression in youth: a meta-analysis of randomized controlled outcome trials.," *PLoS ONE* vol. 10, no. 3, p. e0119895., 2015.
[6]   Y. Perry *et al.*, "Trial for the Prevention of Depression (TriPoD) in final-year secondary students: study protocol for a cluster randomised controlled trial," *Trials [Electronic Resource],* Research Support, Non-U.S. Gov't vol. 16, p. 451, 2015.

[7]   K. K. Fitzpatrick, A. Darcy, and M. Vierhile, "Delivering Cognitive Behavior Therapy to young adults with symptoms of depression and anxiety using a fully automated conversational agent (Woebot): A randomized controlled trial," *JMIR Ment Health,* vol. 4, no. 2, p. e19, Jun 6 2017.

[8]   J. Warren, S. Hopkins, A. Leung, S. Hetrick, and S. Merry, "Building a digital platform for behavioural internvention technology research and deployment," in *Proc 53rd Hawaii International Conference on System Sciences*, 2020.

[9]   R. Williams, "Development of a pilot trial of a chatbot as a digital wellbeing intervention to reduce stress in tertiary students," Master of Science in Psychology thesis, University of Auckland, 2020.

[10] L. Zhou, J. Gao, D. Li, and H.-Y. Shum, "The design and implementation of XiaoIce, an empathetic social chatbot," *Computational Linguistics,* pp. 1-62, 2020.

Healthier Lives, Digitally Enabled
M. Merolli et al. (Eds.)
© 2021 The authors and IOS Press.
This article is published online with Open Access by IOS Press and distributed under the terms
of the Creative Commons Attribution Non-Commercial License 4.0 (CC BY-NC 4.0).
doi:10.3233/SHTI210018

Intended Use of the National Nursing and Midwifery Digital Health Capability Framework

Leanna WOODS [a,1], Elizabeth CUMMINGS [b,c], Naomi DOBROFF [d,e],
Shelley NOWLAN [f], Helen ALMOND [g,h], Paula PROCTER [i], Angela RYAN [a],
Meredith MAKEHAM [a,j], Ken GRIFFIN [k], Julie REEVES [l] and Louise SCHAPER [b]

[a] *Australian Digital Health Agency, Sydney, Australia*
[b] *Australasian Institute of Digital Health, Melbourne, Australia*
[c] *University of Tasmania, Hobart, Australia*
[d] *Australian College of Nursing, Canberra, Australia*
[e] *Monash Health, Melbourne, Australia*
[f] *Clinical Excellence Queensland, Brisbane, Australia*
[g] *Digital Health Cooperative Research Centre, Sydney, Australia*
[h] *Swinburne University of Technology, Melbourne, Australia*
[i] *Sheffield Hallam University, Sheffield, United Kingdom*
[j] *University of Sydney, Sydney, Australia*
[k] *Australian Primary Health Care Nurses Association, Melbourne, Australia*
[l] *Australian Nursing and Midwifery Federation, Melbourne, Australia*

Abstract. To realise the benefits of digital health, the health workforce needs to evolve, adapt and develop their digital proficiency. As the largest workforce in health, nurses and midwives are well positioned to lead as an agile digital healthcare workforce. The objective of this work is to describe how individual nurses and midwives, organisations and education providers could use the newly developed National Nursing and Midwifery Digital Health Capability Framework to build digital health capability. The paper concludes with an international perspective on the framework.

Keywords. digital health, health workforce, capability framework, nursing, midwifery, implementation

1. Introduction

The digitalisation of Australian healthcare settings requires the health workforce to evolve, adapt and build their digital proficiency. This encompasses capability, skills and attitude to operate in a technology-enabled environment [1]. Additionally, the health workforce is increasingly encountering healthcare consumers who expect their healthcare team to be digitally proficient. When implemented correctly, digital health can enhance patient safety and quality, drive workflow and bring cost efficiencies [2, 3].

---

[1] Corresponding Author, Leanna Woods, Australian Digital Health Agency, Level 25, 175 Liverpool St, Sydney, NSW, Australia; E-mail: workforce@digitalhealth.gov.au.

All Australian governments invest significantly in healthcare for their communities. At the present time, governments are focusing on healthcare transformation seeking new and better ways to provide better access to care in an endeavour to address equity gaps. Nurses and midwives are well placed to deliver this care. They partner and mobilise their services with others across the professions and healthcare industry [4]. Key to this transformation is access to information, recording of information and analysing the information for sound clinical decisions in patient care and treatment planning.

Together, nursing and midwifery form the largest healthcare workforce in Australia and as such, they need to lead as an agile digital healthcare workforce. This may be viewed as an individual or organisational responsibility. However, education providers play a significant role in lessening workforce-related pressures on the healthcare system [1]. Educational institutions must take responsibility for adequately preparing our future healthcare workforces by reviewing and adapting their academic programs and embedding digital capabilities. Industry expectations for work-ready graduates and nursing and midwifery program accreditation criteria [5, 6] clearly articulate the need for digital health capabilities training to be embedded within education, ultimately aligning and meeting the demands of the rapidly changing healthcare environment.

The National Nursing and Midwifery Digital Health Capability Framework (the framework) was developed as a practical guide for nurses and midwives to benchmark their current digital health knowledge and skills, and provide a pathway to further their development in this context. Rapid implementation of the framework is supported by the National Digital Health Strategy, which commits to developing a workforce that is able to confidently use digital health technologies and services by 2022 [2].

In the International Year of the Nurse and Midwife, now is the time for the largest workforce in Australia to take the lead in digital health. The purpose of this paper is to provide examples of the potential use of the framework for individual nurses and midwives, organisational managers and education providers.

2. Methods

The development of the framework was led by the Australian Digital Health Agency and the Australasian Institute of Digital Health, in collaboration with a governance group comprising representation from the peak nursing and midwifery bodies in Australia, international and consumer representatives. A draft framework was developed based on national and international evidence and further refined in design workshops. Public consultation across the health sector using an online survey, written submissions and consultation sessions gathered feedback on the draft framework in February and March 2020. The final framework was endorsed in June 2020.

3. The National Nursing and Midwifery Digital Health Capability Framework

The framework describes the digital health capabilities required of nurses and midwives now and into the future. In summary, the framework outlines the core digital health skills, knowledge, and behaviours required for professional practice across five domains:

- Digital Professionalism: Professional standards are maintained in the digital environment

- Leadership and Advocacy: Digital health leadership and advocacy supported by clear policy
- Data and Information Quality: Data quality must be present
- Information-enabled Care: Care must be supported by rigorous data analysis and critical appraisal
- Technology: Technology needs to be understood and used appropriately.

Each domain has three sub-domains which sit within the context of nurses' and midwives' roles, workplace settings, and the professional standards that apply to their practice. Finally, each sub-domain is described by four capability statements. The framework is accompanied by a set of resources and case studies that describe potential examples as suggested through the public consultation.

4. Use of the Framework

Practical examples of how the framework could be used to advance the digital health knowledge and skills for the nursing and midwifery workforce in Australia are proposed below in three different categories: individual nurses and midwives; organisations; and educational providers. The final subsection provides an international perspective on the framework.

4.1. Individual Nurses and Midwives

Primarily, for individuals the framework is intended as a practical guide for nurses and midwives to understand their current digital health knowledge and skills, and provide a pathway to further their professional development. The capability statements, contained within the sub-domains are where users assess their capability level as either formative, intermediate, or proficient. A case study was developed to provide an example of how an individual can use the framework to assess and develop digital health capabilities. Jan is a midwife working in her local public hospital and, with the advent of the COVID-19 pandemic, Jan's workplace has commenced using video-consultations for many antenatal and postnatal visits. Jan has used the framework to find out what additional knowledge and skills she requires to provide care using telehealth (see figure 1). Jan has identified that she has intermediate to proficient skills in most domains, as would be appropriate to her current position. She has noted that she is currently at the foundational level for sub-domains 2.3, 3.3 and 5.2 and, therefore, these are areas where she could expand her knowledge and skills. She can seek professional development opportunities on those topics which can contribute to her annual requirements for continuing professional development.

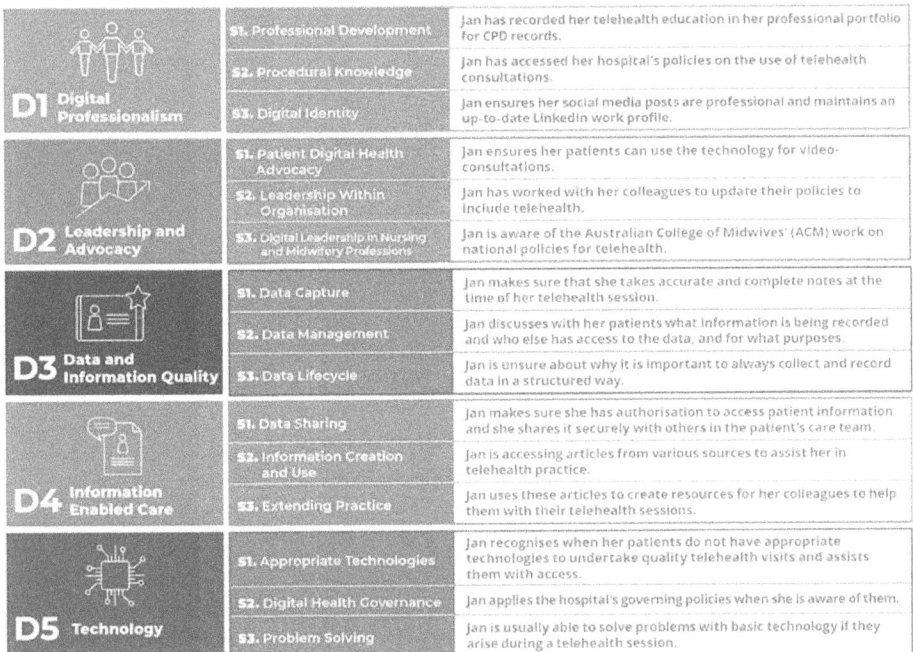

D1 Digital Professionalism	**S1.** Professional Development	Jan has recorded her telehealth education in her professional portfolio for CPD records.
	S2. Procedural Knowledge	Jan has accessed her hospital's policies on the use of telehealth consultations.
	S3. Digital Identity	Jan ensures her social media posts are professional and maintains an up-to-date LinkedIn work profile.
D2 Leadership and Advocacy	**S1.** Patient Digital Health Advocacy	Jan ensures her patients can use the technology for video-consultations.
	S2. Leadership Within Organisation	Jan has worked with her colleagues to update their policies to include telehealth.
	S3. Digital Leadership in Nursing and Midwifery Professions	Jan is aware of the Australian College of Midwives' (ACM) work on national policies for telehealth.
D3 Data and Information Quality	**S1.** Data Capture	Jan makes sure that she takes accurate and complete notes at the time of her telehealth session.
	S2. Data Management	Jan discusses with her patients what information is being recorded and who else has access to the data, and for what purposes.
	S3. Data Lifecycle	Jan is unsure about why it is important to always collect and record data in a structured way.
D4 Information Enabled Care	**S1.** Data Sharing	Jan makes sure she has authorisation to access patient information and she shares it securely with others in the patient's care team.
	S2. Information Creation and Use	Jan is accessing articles from various sources to assist her in telehealth practice.
	S3. Extending Practice	Jan uses these articles to create resources for her colleagues to help them with their telehealth sessions.
D5 Technology	**S1.** Appropriate Technologies	Jan recognises when her patients do not have appropriate technologies to undertake quality telehealth visits and assists them with access.
	S2. Digital Health Governance	Jan applies the hospital's governing policies when she is aware of them.
	S3. Problem Solving	Jan is usually able to solve problems with basic technology if they arise during a telehealth session.

Figure 1. Use of the framework by an individual midwife: A COVID-19 telehealth case study.

4.2. Organisations

The framework has been developed so it can be embedded at a health service or organisational level. The most appropriate nursing and midwifery leaders to undertake this key piece of work are Chief Nursing and Midwifery Information Officers (CNMIOs) as they 'serve as critical links between digital health, organisational change and clinical communities' [7]. Alternatively, a Chief Nursing and Midwifery Officer or similar level nursing and midwifery leader could facilitate this work within a health service context. A flowchart of the steps to assess and improve digital health maturity in an organisation has been developed as a resource to assist with the implementation of this framework (see figure 2).

Prior to commencing the process outlined in the flowchart, organisational governance through the nursing and midwifery professions and commitment to adequate allocation of resources is required. Collaboration between the CNMIO (or equivalent), nursing and midwifery leaders, education teams, digital health team and operational leaders is required, together with engagement and participation from individual nurses and midwives. The flowchart ensures the framework is embedded from an organisational level, commencing with undertaking a subjective assessment of the organisation's level of digital health maturity, the vision and areas for organisational improvement to individual nursing and midwifery staff capability, required resources, and education requirements for staff development. It describes eight discrete but interrelated pieces of work that will need to be undertaken in the order in which they appear. Understanding the outcome of each piece of work is important as this is required to commence the next step. As the flowchart progresses, so will the digital health maturity level of the organisation.

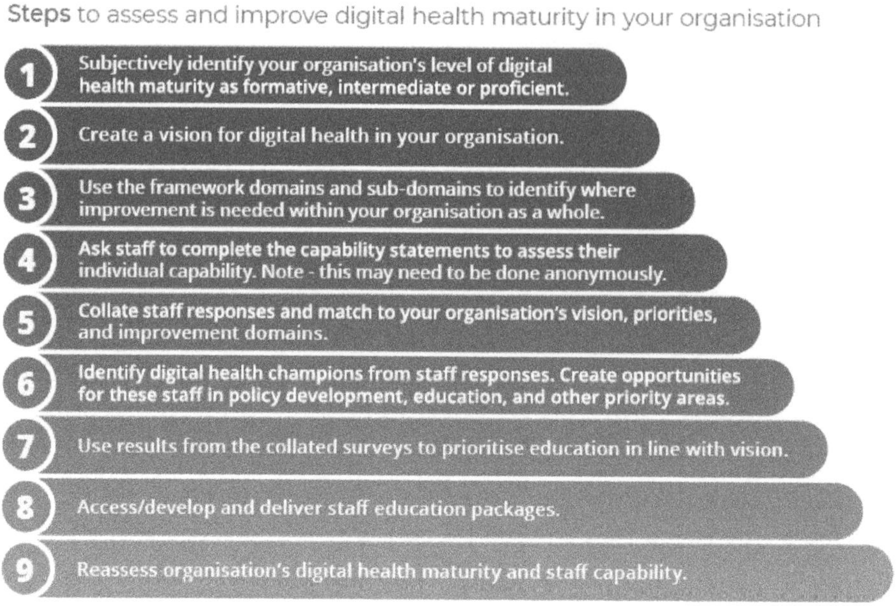

Steps to assess and improve digital health maturity in your organisation

1 Subjectively identify your organisation's level of digital health maturity as formative, intermediate or proficient.

2 Create a vision for digital health in your organisation.

3 Use the framework domains and sub-domains to identify where improvement is needed within your organisation as a whole.

4 Ask staff to complete the capability statements to assess their individual capability. Note - this may need to be done anonymously.

5 Collate staff responses and match to your organisation's vision, priorities, and improvement domains.

6 Identify digital health champions from staff responses. Create opportunities for these staff in policy development, education, and other priority areas.

7 Use results from the collated surveys to prioritise education in line with vision.

8 Access/develop and deliver staff education packages.

9 Reassess organisation's digital health maturity and staff capability.

Figure 2. Use of the framework by an organisation.

The final step is to reassess organisational maturity and staff capability once the other work streams have been completed, ensuring that the flowchart can be revisited to focus on areas for further improvement. Health services that undertake this process and embed the framework will realise a true transition to digital workflows and the associated clinical and professional benefits that support the care provided to communities.

4.3. Education Providers

Embedding the digital health capability framework within a nursing and midwifery educational pathway will not be without its challenges. The largest reported obstacle is lack of resources [8, 9]. However, this is compounded by issues of educator acceptance and knowledge in relation to digital health [8-10]. Successful implementation of any strategy requires recognition by leaders. Nursing and midwifery educational leaders must acknowledge the changing landscape of healthcare delivery. This requires commitment and advocating for nursing and midwifery champions. These champions do not need to be faculty, school or departmental managers, rather enthusiasts with a clear vision and strong commitment to advancing our future workforce.

The champions' focus must be on developing and embedding digital health into the curriculum. This ensures person-centred digital health design, which reflects student learning, clinical partner and accrediting authority requirements. Champions should support and collaborate with industry, ensuring they meet student educational needs. Facilitating all educator learning and timely access to academic digital health technologies (for example, simulated electronic medical and health records, telehealth and mobile health) as well as clinical technologies is a further strategic consideration. Successful embedding and implementation of the framework into curricula is dependent on ensuring the champions are visible within the faculty and supported to drive adoption and utility throughout their program [9].

4.4. International Perspective

In every corner of the world, nurses and midwives are most commonly the primary point of contact for the assessment, delivery, management and evaluation of care to people across all ages. They are the face of care and as such become the information advocate in a complex, multi-professional, multi-dimensional care structure. In many countries there is a growing realisation that digital health capabilities are central to providing continuity of care as we progress further into the 21st century. Development of the framework drew upon the National Health Service Health Education England health and care digital capabilities framework [11] for use by nurses, midwives and allied health professionals. In addition, the UK Royal College of Nursing's publication 'Improving Digital Literacy' [12] was helpful. Both these initiatives are helping to transform the delivery of compassionate care through the use of appropriate supportive technologies.

5. Conclusion

The National Nursing and Midwifery Digital Health Capability Framework clearly identifies a compelling and easy to follow set of attributes that will ensure all Australian nurses and midwives remain at the forefront of care delivery in the information-intensive working environment. The framework is intended to be used by individual nurses and midwives, organisations and education providers. Future work includes empirical evaluation in each setting and the contextualisation of the framework capabilities to other clinical professions.

References

[1] Brunner M, et al. An eHealth Capabilities Framework for Graduates and Health Professionals: Mixed-Methods Study. J Med Internet Res. 2018; 20(5):e10229.
[2] Australian Digital Health Agency. Australia's National Digital Health Strategy: Safe, Seamless and Secure. Sydney: Australian Government; 2017.
[3] Shaw T, Hines M, Kielly-Carroll C. Impact of digital health on the safety and quality of health care. Australian Commission on Safety and Quality in Health Care. Sydney: 2017.
[4] F Hoffmann-La Roche Ltd. Clinical Decision Support, Transforming Complexity into Opportunity: 2020, accessed 31/7/20, www.roche.com/about/business/diagnostics/medical_value/decision-support.htm.
[5] Nursing and Midwifery Board of Australia. Registered nurses standards for practice. Australia: Nursing and Midwifery Board of Australia; 2016.
[6] Nursing and Midwifery Board of Australia. Midwife standards for practice. Australia: Nursing and Midwifery Board of Australia; 2018.
[7] Australian College of Nursing (ACN). Leading digital health transformation: The value of Chief Nursing Information Officer (CNIO) roles – Position Statement. Canberra: ACN; 2019.
[8] Badowski D, et al. Electronic Charting During Simulation: A Descriptive Study. Comput Inform Nurs. 2018; 36(9): 430-437.
[9] Herbert VM, Connors H. Integrating an Academic Electronic Health Record: Challenges and Success Strategies. Comput Inform Nurs. 2016; 34(8): 345-54.
[10] Wilbanks BA, Watts PI, Epps CA. Electronic Health Records in Simulation Education: Literature Review and Synthesis. Simul Healthc. 2018; 13(4): 261-267.
[11] National Health Service / Health Education England (NHS HEE). A Health and Care Digital Capabilities Framework. United Kingdom: NHS HEE; 2017.

[12] Royal College of Nursing (RCN) and NHS HEE. Improving Digital Literacy. United Kingdom: RCN and NHS HEE; 2017.

Healthier Lives, Digitally Enabled
M. Merolli et al. (Eds.)
© 2021 The authors and IOS Press.
This article is published online with Open Access by IOS Press and distributed under the terms
of the Creative Commons Attribution Non-Commercial License 4.0 (CC BY-NC 4.0).

Subject Index

Author Index

Alkhatib, S.	7	Lottridge, D.	92
Almond, H.	106	Louise, S.	32
Archibald, M.	72	Lynch, C.	45
Bain, C.	v	Lythgo, N.	45
Barnett, F.	45	Maeder, A.	51
Beleigoli, A.	72	Makeham, M.	80, 106
Bevens, W.	14	McMillan, P.	72
Bird, S.	45	Mendoza, A.	1
Boyle, J.	32	Merolli, M.	v
Bradford, D.K.	26	Merry, S.	99
Brown, N.J.	20	Milosevic, Z.	58
Buchanan, G.	7	Mudd, A.	72
Cargo, T.	99	Nguyen, A.	20
Chong, C.	92	Nhu, D.	65
Christie, G.	99	Nowlan, S.	106
Cummings, E.	106	Ong, T.Y.	38
Dobroff, N.	106	Pinero De Plaza, M.A.	72
Dobson, R.	92	Procter, P.	106
Feo, R.	72	Pryce, D.	86
Gilligan, A.	65	Rathnayake, K.	38
Gonen, O.	65	Reeves, J.	106
Gough, P.	86	Ryan, A.	80, 106
Gray, K.	1, 14	Schaper, L.K.	v, 106
Griffin, K.	106	Selva-Raj, I.	45
Grobler, M.	7	Shakhatreh, L.	65
Hassanzadeh, H.	32	Sharif Bidabadi, S.	80
Hetrick, S.	99	Shaw, T.	80
Holt-Quick, C.	99	Stasiak, K.	99
Hopkins, S.	99	Taylor, A.	51
Hughes, C.	38	Tieman, J.	51
Hughes, J.A.	20	Tieu, M.	72
Ireland, D.	26	Vu, T.	20
Janmohamed, M.	65	Wang, A.P.	86
Jelinek, G.	14	Wang, S.	7
Kenny, E.	32	Wani, T.A.	1
Khanna, S.	32	Warren, J.	92, 99
Kitson, A.	72	Waycott, J.	7
Kuhlmann, L.	65	Wei Tan, C.	65
Kwan, P.	65	Weiland, T.	14
Lam, V.	38	Westbrook, J.I.	38
Lawless, M.	72	Williams, R.	99
Li, L.	38	Woods, L.	80, 106